THE ART OF WAITING

Also by Belle Boggs

Mattaponi Queen

The Art of Waiting

...

ON FERTILITY, MEDICINE,
AND MOTHERHOOD

Belle Boggs

Graywolf Press

This publication is made possible, in part, by the voters of Minnesota
through a Minnesota State Arts Board Operating Support grant, thanks
to a legislative appropriation from the arts and cultural heritage fund,
and through a grant from the Wells Fargo Foundation Minnesota.
Significant support has also been provided by Target, the McKnight
Foundation, the Amazon Literary Partnership, and other generous con-
tributions from foundations, corporations, and individuals. To these organizations and individuals we offer our heartfelt thanks.

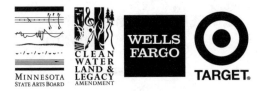

Published by Graywolf Press
250 Third Avenue North, Suite 600
Minneapolis, Minnesota 55401

www.graywolfpress.org

Published in the United States of America

ISBN 978-1-55597-749-8

2 4 6 8 9 7 5 3 1
First Graywolf Printing, 2016

Library of Congress Control Number: 2016931135

Cover design: Kimberly Glyder Design

For my family

CONTENTS

THE ART OF WAITING

The Art of Waiting
...

It's spring when I realize that I may never have children, and around that time the thirteen-year cicadas return, tunneling out of neat, round holes in the ground to shed their larval shells, sprout wings, and fly to the treetops, filling the air with the sound of their singular purpose: reproduction. In the woods where I live, an area mostly protected from habitat destruction, the males' mating song, a vibrating, whooshing, endless hum, a sound at once faraway and up close, makes me feel as though I am living inside a seashell.

Near the river, where the cicadas' song is louder, their discarded larval shells—translucent amber bodies, weightless and eerie—crunch underfoot on my daily walks. Across the river, in a nest constructed near the top of a tall, spindly pine, bald eagles take turns caring for two new eaglets. Turtle hatchlings, snakelets, and ducklings appear on the water. Under my parents' porch, three feral cats give birth in quick succession. And on the news, a miracle pregnancy: Jamani, an eleven-year-old female gorilla, is expecting, the first gorilla pregnancy at the North Carolina Zoo in twenty-two years.

I visit my reproductive endocrinologist's office in May and notice, in the air surrounding the concrete-and-steel hospital complex, a strange absence of sound. There are no tall trees to catch the wind or harbor the cicadas, and on the pedestrian bridge from the parking deck, everyone walks quickly, head down, intent on making their appointments. In the waiting room, I test the leaf surface of a potted ficus with my fingernail and am reassured to find that it is real: green, living.

The waiting room's magazine selection is scanty: a couple of years-old *New Yorkers*, the address labels torn off, and a thick volume of the alarmingly titled *Fertility and Sterility*. On the journal's cover is a small, square photograph of an infant rhesus monkey clasped by an unseen human's hands in a white terry-cloth towel. The monkey wears a startled expression, its dark eyes wide, its mouth forming a tiny pink oval of surprise. A baby monkey hardly seems the thing to put in front of women struggling through the confusion and uncertainties of fertility treatment—*What are those mysterious, grayish blobs on the ultrasound, anyway?*—but, unsure how long I'll wait before my name is called, I reach for the journal. Flipping through, I find another photograph of the monkey and its monkey siblings, and the corresponding article about fertility preservation in human and nonhuman primates exposed to radiation. This monkey's mother, along with twenty other monkeys, was given an experimental drug and exposed to the same kind of radiation administered to women undergoing cancer treatment. On other pages, I find research about mouse testicular cells, peritoneal adhesions in rats, and in vitro fertilization of baboons.

Of course, this research was designed to study human, not animal, infertility. Nonhuman animals don't expose themselves to fertility-compromising radiation therapy; nor do they postpone reproduction, as I have, with years of birth control. Reproducing and ensuring the sexual maturity of offspring is a biological imperative for animals—their success depends on it, and in species after species we see that both males and females will sacrifice everything, their lives, even, to achieve it. But in species with more complex reproductive systems—the animals genetically closest to humans—scientists have documented examples of infertility, hormonal imbalances, endometriosis, and reproductive suppression. *How do they cope?* I wonder, staring at the photo of the baby rhesus monkey, its round, wide-set eyes designed to provoke a maternal response. Do they deal with infertility or the inability to become parents any better—or any differently—than we do?

My name is called, and a doctor I've never met performs a scan of my ovaries. I take notes in a blank book I've filled with four-leaf clovers found on my river walks: *Two follicles? Three? Chance of success 15 to 18 percent.*

On the way out, I steal the journal with the monkey on the cover. Back home, under the canopy of oak and hickory trees, I open the car door, and sound rushes in, louder after its absence. Cicadasong—thousands and thousands of males contracting their internal membranes so that each might find his mate. In Tennessee it gets so bad that a man calls 911 to complain because he thinks it's someone operating machinery.

A few days later, I visit the North Carolina Zoo, where Jamani, the pregnant gorilla, seems unaware of the dozens of extra visitors who have come to see her each day since the announcement of her condition. She shares an enclosure with Acacia, a socially dominant but relatively petite sixteen-year-old female, and Nkosi, a twenty-year-old, 410-pound male. The breeding of captive lowland gorillas is managed by a Species Survival Plan that aims to ensure genetic diversity among captive members of a species. That means adult female gorillas are given birth control pills—the same kind humans take—until genetic testing recommends them for breeding with a male of the same species. Even after clearance, it can take months or years for captive gorillas to conceive. Some never do.

Humans have a long history of imposing various forms of birth control and reproductive technologies on animals, breeding some and sterilizing others. In recent years, we've administered advanced fertility treatments to endangered captive animals such as giant pandas and lowland gorillas. These measures, both high- and low-tech, have come to seem as routine as the management of our own reproduction. We feel responsible when we spay and neuter our cats and dogs, proud when our local zoos release photos of baby animals born of luck and science.

Jamani and Acacia were both brought to the North Carolina Zoo in 2010, after Jamani was recommended for breeding with Nkosi, which was accomplished simply by housing the animals in the same enclosure. The zoo staff confirmed Jamani's pregnancy through an e.p.t. pregnancy test, the kind you can buy at a drugstore.

I ask Aaron Jesue, one of her keepers, if either Jamani or Acacia seems to have registered Jamani's pregnancy, if he or the other keepers have noticed any changes in behavior, but so far the only differences in routine are the increase in zoo visitors to the gorilla exhibit and the many consultations with scientists and zookeepers to help prepare for the birth. "Jamani is still the submissive female," Jesue says. "We'll see if that stays the same."

Many infertile women say that the worst part of the experience is the jealousy they feel toward pregnant women, who seem to be everywhere when you are trying (and failing) to conceive. At the infertility support group I attend, in the basement of another hospital an hour from home, the topic of jealousy and petty hurts frequently begins our conversations.

"I don't mind babies and children, but I hate pregnant women," says one woman, trim and pretty, with a sensible brown bob. "I hate them, and I don't care how that sounds."

So we talk about that for a while: deleting Facebook friends whose frequent status updates document their gestational cycle, steering clear of baby showers and children's birthday parties. We talk about our fears that we will be left out, left behind, while our friends and relatives go about the business of raising their ever-growing families.

The family as a socially isolating unit is an idea not limited to humans. In the wild, infants represent competition for resources, and it is not uncommon for a mother's job to be primarily about hiding and protecting her infants from members of her own species. Jane Goodall observed chimpanzee mothers completely protecting their infants from contact with other, nonsibling chimpanzees for the first five months of life, pulling their infants' hands away when they reached for nearby chimps.

In a marmoset community, the presence of a pregnant female can actually cause infertility in others, though the result is not isolation but rather increased cooperation. Marmosets are tiny South American monkeys that participate in reproductive suppression; typically only one dominant female in a breeding group reproduces, often giving birth to litter after litter before any of the others has a chance. This is accomplished through behavior—some females simply do not mate—and also through a specialized neuroendocrine response to the perception of subordination, which, like the pill, inhibits ovarian follicular development and ovulation. Some never get their chance but remain in the submissive, nonbreeding category all their lives.

Marmosets make their nests in rain-forest canopies and live in groups of three to fifteen, feeding on spiders, insects, and small vertebrates. Peaceful cooperation is remarkable among marmosets, particularly in regard to infant care. All group members over five months of age—male, female, dominant, subordinate—participate, and a dominant female will allow her offspring to be carried by other group members from the first day of life. Scientists have speculated that this dependence on helpers—marmosets usually give birth to twins—is the reason for behavioral and hormonal reproductive suppression. The phenomenon of suppression occurs both in the wild and in captivity.

Occasionally a subordinate female will reproduce, although

her infant has a diminished chance of survival. One reason is the practice of infanticide, which researchers have observed multiple times in the wild (more frequently, the tiny infants just disappear). Infanticide most commonly occurs when a subordinate female gives birth during the pregnancy of the dominant female, who is often the attacker. Despite the apparent brutality of such a system, it does not seem to diminish social relationships or cooperation among the marmosets.

Sometimes cooperation is so extensive that it becomes difficult for researchers to establish which female is the biological mother. In one instance, recorded by Leslie Digby in Brazil in 1991, two adult females gave birth to twins in the same week. Less than a month later, two of the infants had disappeared, but because both mothers continued to nurse both surviving infants, it was impossible to tell which female was the biological mother or "even whether those that disappeared were members of a single litter," according to Digby's report.

Like ours, the animal world is full of paradoxical examples of gentleness, brutality, and suffering, often performed in the service of reproduction. Female black widow spiders devour their partners after a complex and delicate mating dance. Bald eagle parents, who mate for life and share the responsibility of rearing young, will sometimes look on impassively as the stronger eaglet kills its sibling. At the end of their life cycle, after swimming thousands of miles in salt water, Pacific salmon swim up their natal, freshwater streams to spawn while the freshwater decays their flesh. Animals will do whatever it takes to ensure reproductive success.

For humans, *whatever it takes* has come to mean in vitro fertilization (IVF), a procedure developed in the 1970s that involves the hormonal manipulation of a woman's cycle followed by the harvest and fertilization of her eggs, which are transferred as embryos to her uterus. More than 5 million babies worldwide have been born through IVF, which has become a multibillion-dollar industry.

"Test-tube baby," says another woman at the infertility support group, a young ER doctor who has given herself five at-home inseminations and is thinking of moving on to IVF. "I really hate that term. It's a baby. That's all it is." She has driven seventy miles to talk to seven other women about the stress and isolation of infertility.

In the clinics, they call what the doctors and lab technicians do ART—assisted reproductive technology—softening the idea of the test-tube baby, the lab-created human. Art is something human, social, nonthreatening. Art does not clone or copy, but creates. It is often described as priceless, timeless, healing. It is far from uncommon to spend large amounts of money on art. It's an investment.

All of these ideas are soothing, whether we think them through or not, just as the experience of treating infertility, while often painful and undignified, soothes as well. For the woman, treating infertility is about nurturing her body, which will hopefully produce eggs and a rich uterine lining where a fertilized egg could implant. All of the actions she might take in a given month—abstaining from caffeine and alcohol, taking Clomid or Femara, injecting herself with Gonal-f or human chorionic gonadotropin, charting her temperature and cervical mucus on a specialized calendar—are essentially maternal, repetitive, and self-sacrificing. In online message boards where women gather to talk about their Clomid cycles and inseminations and IVF cycles, a form of baby talk is used to discuss the organs and cells of the reproductive process. Ovarian follicles are "follies," embryos are "embies," and frozen embryos—the embryos not used in an IVF cycle that are frozen for future tries—are "snowbabies." The frequent ultrasounds given to women in a treatment cycle, which monitor the growth of follicles and the endometrial lining, are not unlike the ultrasounds of pregnant women in the early stages of pregnancy. There is a wand, a screen, and something growing.

And always: something more to do, something else to try. It doesn't take long, in an ART clinic, to spend tens of thousands of dollars on tests, medicine, and procedures. When I began to wonder why I could not conceive, I said the most I would do was read a book and chart my temperature. My next limit was pills: I would take them, but no more than that. Next was intra-uterine insemination, a less-expensive, low-tech procedure that requires no sedation. Compared with the women in my support group, women who leave the room to give themselves injections in the hospital bathroom, I'm a lightweight. Often during their discussions of medications and procedures, I have no idea what they're talking about, and part of the reason I attend each month is to listen to their horror stories. I'm hoping to detach from the process, to see what I could spare myself if I gave up.

But after three years of trying, it's hard to give up. I know that it would be better for the planet if I did (if infinitesimally so), better for me, in some ways, as a writer. Certainly giving up makes financial sense. In my early twenties, when I saw such decisions as black or white, right or wrong, I would have felt it was selfish and wasteful to spend thousands of dollars on un-necessary medical procedures. Better, the younger me would have argued, to donate the money to an orphanage or a children's hospital. Better to adopt.

The thirty-four-year-old me has careful but limited savings, knows how difficult adoption is, and desperately wants her body to work the way it is supposed to.

A large part of the pressure and frustration of infertility is the idea that fertility is normal, natural, and healthy, while infertility is rare and unnatural and means something is wrong with you. It's not usually a problem you anticipate; from the time we are very young, we are warned and promised that pregnancy will one day happen. At my support group, someone always says how surprised she is to be there.

My parents married in their early twenties and moved to the country to live on a farm and raise a family. It took them thirteen months to conceive me, and my mother says that during those months of waiting she thought she had been ruined by her previous years of birth control. That's how she put it— *ruined*—as if the rest of her working body, her strong back, her artist's hands, her quick wit, did not matter.

Although I married almost as young as my mother—I was twenty-six—it never occurred to me to have children right away. In my first year of marriage, I was teaching writing workshops to kindergarteners in Brooklyn, and at the beginning of the year I remember drawing and labeling a diagram of my bedroom on a big pad of paper while my students worked in their own notebooks. Daniel, a bright and charming five-year-old, pointed at the drawing of my bed. "Why are there *two* pillows?" he asked. "One for me, and one for my husband," I said. He gasped. "You're going to have a baby!" I laughed and shook my head. "I'm too young to have a baby," I said. On parent-teacher night I realized that Daniel's own parents were younger than I was.

Three years later, I invited a public health nurse to speak to a group of fifth graders I was teaching in North Carolina. The subject of her talk was "your changing bodies," a reliable source of giggles, but the nurse, a beautiful and soft-spoken woman who happened to be blind, brought a hushed seriousness to the talk. She angled her face upward so that her lecture took on the air of prayer, and she handled the plastic anatomical models of the vagina and uterus reverently. "Your bodies are miracles," she told the girls in a separate session. "They are built to have babies. That is the reason for menstruation, the reason for the changes your body will go through."

"Your brains are miracles, too," I told them later. "Bigger

miracles than your uteruses. You don't have to have a baby if you don't want to." But my words sounded feeble and undignified next to the nurse's serene pronouncement.

I'm always surprised when my students, boys and girls alike, from kindergarteners to high school seniors, talk about the children they will have someday. "My kids won't act like that," they say, eyeing an unruly class on a field trip. Or, worriedly, "I bet I'll have all boys. What will I do with all boys?" It seems far more common for them to imagine the children they might have than the jobs they might do or the places they might live.

Perhaps I shouldn't be surprised. Perhaps imagining ourselves as parents is not only the expression of a biological drive but essential to understanding the scope of our lives, who we are and who we might become. For years I have dealt with a dread of old age and death by reminding myself, *I have not yet given birth.* I can imagine the moment clearly—my husband is there next to me, my parents are waiting to meet their grandchild—and the fact that it hasn't happened (always, it is at least nine months away) reassures me that some new stage of life is still to come. I'm not sure when people started asking me if I have children—a couple of years ago, I think. "Not yet," I always say.

Tillie Olsen's groundbreaking feminist *Silences* includes a chapter titled "The Damnation of Women," on the choice many women writers made between work and children. Olsen writes that it is not until the twentieth century that "an anguish, a longing to have children, breaks into expression. In private diaries and letters only." Her selections from Virginia Woolf's diaries in particular are extraordinary for their candor and pain. Woolf, who never had children, struggled with the idea of that loss for more than a decade, writing:

> *. . . and all the devils came out—heavy black ones—to be*
> *29 & unmarried—to be a failure—childless—insane too,*
> *no writer . . .*

She seems to have conflated the failure to reproduce with artistic failure, though she is only two years away from finishing her first novel. In her thirties, still childless, just a few years from writing *Mrs. Dalloway,* she again writes of "having no children" and "failing to write well" in the same sentence. At forty-four, she describes the dread she feels observing her sister's life as an artist and mother:

> *Let me watch the wave rise. I watch. Vanessa. Children. Failure. Yes. Failure. Failure. The wave rises.*

It is only after embracing her writing as an "anchor" that she makes peace with her childlessness:

> *I can dramatise myself as a parent, it is true. And perhaps I have killed the feeling instinctively; or perhaps nature does.*

Because we spend much of our young lives imagining ourselves as parents, it isn't surprising that even the strongest of us let the body's failure become how we define ourselves. But life, which gives us other things to do, tells us otherwise. The feeling of grief subsides; we think through our options and make choices. We work, travel, find other ways to be successful. After completing *The Waves,* at forty-eight, Woolf writes of a feeling of intoxication that comes from writing well:

> *Children are nothing to this.*

I'm no Virginia Woolf, but on occasion, after a good stretch of writing or time spent happily alone, I've had that feeling. It's thrilling, like taking a drug or riding a bicycle down a steep hill. Probably it isn't that different from the feeling a new mother has, looking at her child. *Not yet,* I've thought, suddenly protective of my time, my privacy, my freedom.

I once asked my father, "Does having kids really squash all your dreams?"

He thought for a minute. "Yep," he said. "And it takes all your money too."

On the North Carolina Zoo's Facebook page, Jamani's keepers have posted a video of her latest sonogram. In a practiced pose, Jamani stands upright in an indoor room, clutching the steel grate that separates her from the zoo's staff. Her belly is accessible through a small gap in the grate. Humans and gorillas are so closely related that staff members wear hospital masks to protect themselves and Jamani from viruses.

"Hands up, hands up," one zookeeper says, clicking a training noisemaker while another keeper feeds her from a platter of vegetables. "Belly." Jamani does not move her hands, but the keeper repeats the commands every few seconds. She is praised for her compliance, and the black-and-white image of her baby, looking not unlike the human sonograms I've seen on Facebook, appears on the veterinarian technician's laptop. I've watched it a dozen times, studying Jamani's face for clues to her comprehension.

"So neat!" comments one poster beneath the link.

"She is doing great," says another.

"The Baby is a cutie already," writes another.

Waiting in the outdoor enclosure during the filming, childless Acacia must be sitting on her haunches, chomping lettuce or carrots, oblivious to the fuss being made over Jamani, unaware of the fuss to come. Part of the reason for the attention from the media, from veterinarians, and from zoos across the country is the pregnancy's rarity among captive gorillas, and its uncertainty. In 2010, only six successful gorilla births were recorded in American zoos, and even when infants are born healthy, there's the chance that the mother will reject her young. If this happens, Jamani's keepers plan for Acacia to take over as a surrogate. Meanwhile, Acacia mates with Nkosi regularly, though she has taken birth control pills since 2001 and will remain on birth control until the gorilla Species Survival Plan determines that she is compatible with Nkosi. She may never conceive, but, according to her keepers, she seems content.

Nonhuman animals wait without impatience, without a deadline, and I think that is the secret to their composure. Reproductively mature for more than half her life, Acacia waits without knowing she is waiting. The newly hatched cicadas will wait underground for another thirteen years. The submissive marmoset who declines sex, or whose ovaries fail to produce mature follicles, waits and waits—maybe forever.

Though infertile women are aware of the passing of months and years—marked by charts, appointments, prescriptions, and pregnancy tests—we have something animals lack, which is the conscious possibility of a new purpose, a sense of self not tied to reproduction. I think it comes to us eventually, as Woolf suggests, but perhaps knowing that it comes, and understanding infertility as a natural, perhaps even useful phenomenon, can provide us with a measure of peace. Marmoset communities would not survive without their reproductively suppressed, caretaking females. Had Virginia Woolf been a mother, she might not have given us *Mrs. Dalloway, To the Lighthouse, A Room of One's Own, The Waves.*

The cicadas stop their noise at the end of May. The adults are dead—eaten by other animals, worn out from their reproductive frenzy—and their wings litter the ground that will protect and nurture their young.

The silence is startling at first—I step outside each morning expecting to hear that seashell sound—but it's also a relief. I wait for some other wave.

Baby Fever

...

In the long opening sequence of Joel and Ethan Coen's *Raising Arizona,* Hi, a petty criminal moderately reformed by the stern love of a policewoman named Ed, explains the unselfish origins of his wife's desire for a baby: "Her point was that there was too much love and beauty for just the two of us," he narrates over a shot of the two of them enjoying a magnificent desert sunset. "Every day we kept a child out of the world was a day he might later regret having missed." They work at it, and work at it, as Ed posts aspirational photos of babies—round faced, adorable, grinning, crying—around their trailer. Sometime later a doctor confirms what they'd begun to fear—Ed's womb was "a rocky place" where Hi's "seed could find no purchase." After looking into Hi's past, an adoption agency rejects them—go figure— and they fall into depression. Ed loses her job and can barely dress herself, the trailer is a shambles—the "pizazz" goes out of their lives, as Hi puts it—until they kidnap Nathan Junior, one of the Arizona quints born to wealthy owners of an unpainted furniture empire, to raise as their own.

Before Richard and I got married, we agreed that *Raising Arizona* was our favorite movie—funny, tender, slapstick. Between us we could recite most of it from memory, and one year while we were living in Los Angeles, we dressed up as Hi and Ed for Halloween. There's a photograph of us in a shoe box

17

somewhere, Richard wearing a Hawaiian shirt with a stocking pulled over his head and a package of Huggies under his arm. I'm in a police uniform with a baby doll on my hip. Hardly anyone recognized our costumes on Santa Monica Boulevard, a Halloween thoroughfare crowded with superheroes and strippers, but we didn't mind. We saw something of ourselves in those characters—not in their situation, but in their personas, the way they interact with the rest of the world and the pure devotion they have to each other. Richard, like Hi, was articulate and deadpan and love struck. I was more like Ed, a high-minded stickler for the rules.

It took years for us to try for a critter of our own, so many that by the time we first suspected trouble we didn't remember the costumes we wore, or the conflict at the heart of our favorite film. There were too many other things to think about: how we would pay for expensive fertility treatments, when we would say "enough," whether to adopt or foster a child and how we would pay for that, too. When we finally remembered what more we had in common with Hi and Ed—it was Richard who pointed it out—the realization felt less bitter and more inevitable, fated. This is what it means to be people who want something very much but can't have it. Why shouldn't we be those people?

My desire had manifested itself differently from Ed's—I can remember wiping away spots of blood a few months after stopping the Pill and thinking, *I must be pregnant.* (I'd read that late-cycle spotting was a sign of an embryo's implantation.) In the same moment I had a panicked sense of all I hadn't done: publish a book, establish my career, travel. I wasn't pregnant; the spotting was actually a symptom of my infertility, masked for so many cycles by birth control. After another year we sought medical help. By then, instead of posting baby pictures, I bookmarked websites about assisted reproduction, about adoption, about foster care. I agonized over my basal body temperature, took pills that made me weepy, paid for medical treatments with a slim chance of success. If someone had told me, "In five years you will have a baby," I would have been fine to wait those five years; I would have been grateful to have them, in fact, and would have gotten busy with some of my other goals.

But no one could tell me that—the problem with infertility is that it is not a patient, serene kind of waiting, not a simple delay in your plans; it happens for many of us in the context of consuming struggle, staggering expense, devastating loss. It's five (or eight, or ten) years of trying and failing, which erodes any feelings of confidence or anticipation of a positive outcome.

Richard and I stopped our first rounds of treatment after two years, the most difficult time I'd ever experienced. But stronger than my sadness over our failed cycles was the feeling of relief to be done with medication and monthly disappointment. For a while I consoled myself with the benefits of childlessness. I won a fellowship and cut back my teaching hours. I wrote half of one novel, then all of another one. I sat in on a class in evolutionary biology at Duke University, feverishly taking notes on extraordinary examples of self-sacrificing mating displays and behavior in birds and other animals:

The blue-backed manakin practices his mating dance for eight or nine years before debuting it in front of females. Male barn swallows with long tail feathers are more vulnerable to predators, but also more attractive to females. Australian redback spiders are so intent their offspring survive that males catapult themselves into the jaws of their mates immediately after copulation, providing extra nutritional resources for the female and her young.

I wanted to feel lucky—to be human, free, unencumbered by blind instinct. I had no children, but look what I could do: drive thirty miles on a Monday morning to sit in a lecture hall and take notes studded with exclamation points and question marks, to feel the pleasurable jolts of new information landing in my brain.

Still, some days I felt like Ed in the days before she kidnapped Nathan Junior: bereft and lonely, consumed by longing. "I don't feel like myself," I remember telling Richard. More accurately, I felt split in two. The person I had hoped to become was torn away, leaving only the person I had always been.

The first evolutionary psychologist, Edward Westermarck, suggested in his 1891 book, *The History of Human Marriage,* that humans share a universal "child-bearing instinct." Sexologist Havelock Ellis scoffed at this, claiming that instinct obviously manifests itself through the sexual impulse—nature doesn't need two drivers of reproduction. That would be redundant, and redundancy is rare in evolution. Westermarck removed his claim from future editions of his book.

The existence of an innate human desire to reproduce is still debated among scientists. "We are genetically predisposed to seek sexual relations," observed eminent obstetrician and reproductive scientist Malcolm Potts, more recently. "It is possible to find many people who want sex but who do not want to have children, but there is no significant group of heterosexuals who want children but do not wish to have sex." (I can think of some: infertile couples exhausted by the romance-killing phenomenon of timed intercourse, but they probably don't count.) Humans are unquestionably driven by sex: we have it even when women are not fertile, and frequent sex, unrelated to estrus, tends to bond us in relatively stable pairings, which may make raising our children easier but is not the reason we have it. Given our relatively brief period of fertility each month, our long stretches of infertility during pregnancy and lactation, and the low implantation rate of human embryos, conception without birth control is merely "a probabilistic event" and not the result of conscious trying, according to Potts.

Further argument for a low conscious desire to reproduce: since the advent of reliable contraceptives and safe abortions, we've used them. In America, 62 percent of reproductive-age women use some form of birth control; at current rates, 30 percent of American women will have had abortions by their forty-fifth birthdays. Before we had birth control, women controlled their birth rate using various forms of folk medicine meant to induce abortion. Humans are an extraordinarily successful species, yet we have few children—an average of 2.5 children per woman worldwide, fewer in developed countries. Studies of preliterate societies reveal a higher fertility rate, but not extraordinarily so—4 to 6 children born to each woman, with about half of the children dying before the advent of sexual maturity.

Our relatively low fertility rate works out well for our big-brained yet helpless infants. From birth they take an unparalleled amount of care, and we continue to care for them—feeding them, tending them, keeping them safe, and teaching them survival and social skills—well into (and sometimes beyond) their second decade of life. But this is not necessarily a sign that we are less driven than our mammalian forebears to pass along our genes. Instead, reproductive ecologists insist, it's evidence that we are programmed to prioritize quality over quantity, investing a great deal of nurturing and resources on each child.

Perhaps a more compelling argument for the reproductive drive (not just the sex drive) is the behavior of both sexes around the time of ovulation. Though they'll have sex anytime, men find women nearing estrus more attractive than at other times during their cycle—they smell better, have a more appealing hip-to-waist ratio, have softer, more symmetrical features, and are perceived to be wittier and more creative. Women, for their part, dress more provocatively and more fashionably at estrus; maybe we work harder at witty conversation, too. Reflecting both male preference and female effort, a study found that women employed as lap dancers in Albuquerque make twice as much in tips during their most fertile time.

Mate selection is also influenced by expressions of child longing or, at least, child friendliness. By playing enthusiastically with children or desirously grabbing babies' toes, knitting layette blankets or tiny sweaters, or otherwise appearing sympathetic to children, men and women alike demonstrate that they are good potential partners, capable of putting in the long years of care required by human offspring. Though Richard and I were a long time from trying when we wore our Hi and Ed costumes, it's likely that we each read positive caretaking traits into our joint choice of costume. I remember an us-against-the-world connectedness as we strolled down Santa Monica Boulevard; I enjoyed the spectacle of Richard with the ridiculous panty on his head, the heft of plastic Nathan Junior against my hip. Two months later, we were engaged.

Child-longing—this is what I had during the height of my experience with assisted reproduction and what I am trying to account for, explain, trace back to its beginnings. More than anything, this is what I wanted: to hold a child of my own, be clung to in that way that primate infants have—legs wrapped around my middle, a hand in my hair and another on my arm. In the same way that it's difficult to imagine the manakin practicing eight years solely to have sex, the theories of mate selection we learned about in evolutionary biology class seemed to trivialize my desire for a child, which felt like my own, independent pursuit. Not an impulse in the service of another impulse, but something pure.

Human child-longing goes by different names, depending where you live. The English call women afflicted by this condition broody, a term borrowed from the henhouse. (Broody hens are the ones who won't rest or roost but sit constantly on a clutch of eggs, sometimes plucking out their breast feathers to keep the eggs warm.) Americans, perpetual taskmasters, say that the biological clock is ticking. In Scandinavia they call it baby fever, a widely observed condition that manifests itself as everything from a generalized wishing for a child to a delirious, aching sickness. Finnish family sociologist Anna Rotkirch studied the phenomenon and its implications for her field—do we have an evolved desire to have babies?—by asking readers of a major Finnish newspaper to write to her about their experiences with baby fever. She received 106 responses from women and 7 from men. The male responses were too few, general, or impersonal to be used in her study (two of their responses complained of suffering caused by the "baby feverish" women in their lives), but the women's letters were intimate and detailed, with many describing the fever as an inescapable, unbidden, and often inconvenient fact of life.

> *I was infected when I took a six-week-old baby in my arms . . . It was an all-encompassing desire for a child, without any trace of common sense and ignoring the consequences. Actually a very agonising experience.*

Many of the respondents recalled dreams as the first sign of baby fever:

> *About ten years ago strange things started happening. As I turned 28, I started having dreams about children almost every night. I had a restless feeling all the time, just as if my womb was demanding something I did not agree with. I started thinking about having a child, although I knew that I did not want it under any circumstances.*

In the same way that illness can rack the body, baby fever is painful and all encompassing:

*I was 25 years old when it hit. And it really HIT me, the
feeling caused by baby fever was unlike anything I had
experienced earlier in life. It was something totally biological, because I did not experience any outer pressure, on the
contrary, my parents for instance stressed that I should have
a good job before starting a family. I had been dating my
boyfriend for six years, we were both studying and the idea
was to graduate quickly and start making a career, and
children were not part of that constellation yet for a long
time to come.*

For those who cannot act on the impulse to have children—
Finnish people place a high value on education and becoming
settled in a career first—the longing grows even stronger:

*My baby fever has become uncontrollable. I have dreams
about babies all the time. I have to touch baby clothes in
stores. I ponder the alternative of ecological nappies. On
the streets I smile at children I do not know. In every single
long-term plan, I take into account our future children.
Sometimes I [lie] awake at night and feel a huge longing,
which starts from my womb and radiates to all parts of my
body. A physical, compelling, painful need to be pregnant. If
somebody had earlier tried to describe such a feeling to me, I
would probably have rolled my eyes, encouraged her to climb
out of the swamp of motherhood myth and get a life. We
have agreed to try to have children in a year or two. I count
the days.*

When prolonged, either by infertility or other circumstances,
baby fever can cause the opposite effect—instead of feeling
drawn to babies and young children and the baby aisles of
stores, sufferers begin avoiding places where they'll encounter
reminders of what they cannot have. They grow alienated from

pregnant friends or friends with children, sometimes ending relationships that become too painful.

Rotkirch describes baby fever as "an emotion which may be typical for societies where women have many choices." It appears to be heightened, she says, by proximity to children and especially babies, as well as—unfortunately, for some of us—the presence of obstacles. What makes Rotkirch's study notable is not that it describes women longing for children but that it includes women who have always wanted children (the natural nurturers) as well as those who have not; women from both categories confess to the experience of baby fever and report it as an unbidden, surprising phenomenon that often works against their other goals. Finland is a low-fertility country that promotes individualism and education; more than half of Rotkirch's subjects were born between 1960 and 1980, when these values were firmly established. Yet the respondents wrote candidly, passionately, about baby clothes and diapers and the particular smell of babies' heads, all the traditional material and physical trappings of infancy and motherhood.

The idea to study child-longing evolved out of Rotkirch's own experience. In her late thirties, already a mother of two and at a productive time in her career, she felt an intense desire to have a third child. Even though she and her husband agreed for a variety of reasons that they would stop at two, her baby fever only increased, and she eventually became pregnant. While on maternity leave, she decided to look into baby fever and was surprised to find nothing in the scientific literature supporting her suspicions, only reports of babies with fevers.

"It was funny to me, [someone] who tries to combine women's/ gender studies and feminism with evolutionary psychology, that both these disciplines vehemently DENIED there could even be such a thing," Rotkirch told me over email. "Feminists said patriarchy lures women to want babies, and evolutionary psychologists said it is a mistake to think people want babies (since they want sex)."

But she thought there was something to her idea that baby fever is an emotion in its own right, even though she admits that for some, this line of research appears less serious than her other work, which investigates family and fertility decisions in a more quantitative way. Rotkirch suspected that an intense desire for a child was not merely a social construction but something deeper, biological, that could answer important questions about why people want to have children at all and whether low-fertility countries would continue to see birthrates decline (her study of baby fever suggests the current birthrate is somewhat stable).

That doesn't mean that all women will experience this phenomenon or that women who don't should take it as a sign that they shouldn't plan to have a family. But it does illuminate the experiences of people like me, who have been overcome by a desire for a baby but have obstacles in our path. For us, baby fever could have the function of pushing us to make a decision, or the practical use of explaining our irrational pursuit of an elusive goal.

> *It had come over me quite suddenly, in my mid-twenties, when I was working for* Vogue, *a tidal surge. Once this surge hit I saw babies wherever I went. I followed their carriages on the street. I cut their pictures from magazines and tacked them to the wall next to my bed. I put myself to sleep by imagining them: imagining holding them, imagining the down on their heads, imagining the soft spots at their temples, imagining the way their eyes dilated when you looked at them.*

That's not a response to Rotkirch's study but an excerpt from Joan Didion's *Blue Nights,* her memoir of adoptive motherhood and grief. It's interesting to me how Didion's exacting, often detached writing style here mirrors the perplexed confessions elicited by Rotkirch's questionnaire, and also how the Finnish respondents, in describing something both private and deeply felt, write almost as eloquently as Didion. I sent Rotkirch the passage, and she wrote back that it was "unsettling," so close to some of her subjects' written memories that she wondered at first if they'd read *Blue Nights* (in fact it was published after she collected their responses).

I cut their pictures from magazines and tacked them to the wall: that's also exactly what Ed does.

My mother had it, bad, at a time when baby fever, or the maternal instinct, or the need to nurture—whatever you want to call it—was unpopular, and she was poor and young, making her living painting murals and signs and doing odd artist jobs: teaching embroidery to prison inmates, painting dancers' bodies at discotheques. None of her girlfriends had kids. They had exquisitely long hair and willowy limbs, freewheeling boyfriends and trips to California; they had tattoos and abortions, but no kids, and they weren't alone. Individualism, feminism, and free love sounded better to many people in the 1970s—more glamorous, more fun, more free, even more responsible—than the previous generation's ideal of a big, suburb-dwelling family.

My mother was a hippie, but she didn't want free love and freedom—she wanted to marry my father, who looked to her like Jesus (my dad was a hippie too), and have kids with him (falling in love, Rotkirch found, is one of the primary triggers for baby fever). That was always a calculation for her—do I want this person to father my kids? My dad was smart and strong and independent and kind; she valued all those things and wanted them for her children. Plus, he was handsome. That helped too.

They were married in my grandparents' backyard in April 1973, when the azaleas were blooming. The blossoms are pink and white, blurry and exuberant, in the backgrounds of their wedding photos; my mother, twenty-three years old, wears a lacy blue dress and a white veil; my dad, twenty-two, wears a brown tuxedo with a ruffled shirt. A few months after they were married, my mom rode her bike with a friend across the Lee Bridge in Richmond to a secondhand store that sold bags full of clothes for a dollar a piece. Amid the heaps of prairie dresses and blue jeans she found a tiny pair of overalls, bright blue with red buttons and lined in soft, red flannel. She tucked them into her dollar bag, took them home, and embroidered them with a mouse, a smiling moon, and stars.

Nigel, my cousin, was the first to wear the overalls, which have been passed around among family and close friends for years. "They were for *you*," my mother told me when I asked if she'd embroidered them for him. She was jealous of her flighty younger brother, who'd gotten his girlfriend pregnant by accident, and it pained her to wait even the thirteen months it took her to conceive me. By the time I was born, Nigel had grown out of them. My brother wore them a few years later, then my mother's friend Donna's children and my two younger cousins. Another friend of my mother's, a woman who became pregnant by happy surprise in her forties, borrowed them for a year for her daughter. Then my mother took them back, wrapped them in tissue, and stored them in her cedar chest for me.

Though I had neither designs on becoming pregnant nor any inclination to browse baby clothes at age twenty-three—no baby fever yet—I knew that I wanted those overalls, and all they represented, someday. By now they are so faded they're almost white, as soft as a pillowcase. I remember my mother getting them out and showing them to me anytime we sorted through her most precious things—*Someday these will be my grandbaby's*—and feeling attracted to the idea that I would be part of my family's legacy through child rearing. No matter how far away I moved, or how different my life might be from my parents', I would do the same things my mother had: sing the same songs, read the same books, play the same games. I would grow closer to my mother but also to my childhood self. As Jennifer Senior points out in *All Joy and No Fun,* children "create wormholes in time," offering us a chance to experience our own childhoods, which so many of us idealize through memory, all over again.

Like a manakin, I had practiced for years. Not long after I grew out of those overalls, I was buttoning them onto baby dolls that I fed from bottles, bathed, and pushed around the yard in a stroller. My first job was babysitting for three brothers; we played indoor hide-and-seek and slid around their sparsely furnished McMansion in our socks. I adopted a dog a year after moving out of my parents' house, when I was a sophomore in college, and used him as an excuse to spend long weekend afternoons at the river, a childhood pastime. My first job out of graduate school was teaching at an elementary school in Brooklyn, where I read stories, taught math and writing, painted pictures, wiped noses. We weren't allowed to hug the children, but they could hug or lean against us. I stood still as a tree (the recommended stance) when I remembered, but I hugged them back just as often.

By *practiced,* I don't mean to say that those experiences were meant only to prepare me for the more important task of raising my own child. I loved my terrier, despite his predilection for insane barking and occasional biting, and I loved my students too. Those activities—caretaking, nurturing—are valuable in their own right and a contribution to my life and (I hope) the lives of those I cared for. But my attraction to being a caretaker felt even then like it was in service of something else—a longer, more profound relationship than the borrowed time I spent with first graders. It also felt like something I couldn't help very much.

If biology and genetics influenced my mother's—and my own— susceptibility to baby fever, culture may have cemented it.

Aside from possibly imparting a genetic proceptive tendency, my grandmother almost certainly raised my mother with the expectation that she would one day have her own family; my mother raised my brother and me with the same idea. Pronatalism is the idea that parenting is a normalizing rite of passage, something we must each go through to achieve full status as productive, responsible adults; it gets expressed in political propaganda, in the media and popular culture, in art and literature, and—perhaps most powerfully—in the attitudes of our own families. It works on us whether we realize it or not, validating our choices or making us feel like outsiders.

The desirability of biological children is coded into most of the world's major religions and into humanity's first lasting artistic expressions. The god of the Hebrew Bible commanded Adam and Eve to be fruitful and multiply; Islam encourages procreation as one of the purposes of marriage and even frowns upon monasticism and celibacy. Hindus believe that children are gifts and a reflection of karma. The earliest known works of figurative art, created some thirty-five thousand years ago, are sculptures of women with absent or masked faces and exaggerated sexual characteristics: wide hips, large breasts, prominent vulvas. They are thought to be fertility goddesses.

American expressions of pronatalism date back to colonial times, when preachers used their sermons to praise mothers with large families and nudge the slackers to get busy—the average female colonist had about eight children, though only four would live to adulthood. Pronatalism has been a means of control, of encouraging the right people to have children for the benefit of the powerful. Until they were seen as profitable breeding factories, enslaved African women were discouraged from having children in America. But white, middle-class or prosperous Americans were frequently told it was their duty to have as many children as possible—during the nineteenth century, to drive out Native Americans and populate the western territories; and in the early twentieth century, to avoid "race suicide." The idea that some people should have children while others should not inspired and popularized the American eugenics movement.

Pronatalism peaked during the post–World War II years of prosperity and conformism—that's one reason there are so many baby boomers—and declined as Generation Xers were being born (which is one reason there are so few of us, relatively speaking). From 1941 to 1960, 0 percent of Americans considered no children the ideal family size; childless people were seen as selfish deviants or pitiable losers, while family men and women were patriotic heroes. By the time my mother was rummaging through thrift bins for baby clothes, American culture—thanks largely to feminism and environmentalism—had finally made room for child-free lifestyles. Child-free women and couples were given voice in traditional media, and organizations such as the Childfree Network provided support for the voluntarily childless. RESOLVE: The National Infertility Association, founded in 1974, offered support for infertile women and men and a replacement for the narrative of the pitiable outsider.

Though the fertility rate has remained relatively stable since the less-prolific 1970s, cultural expressions of pronatalism have made a comeback. Television programs once again exalt the procreative, from reality shows such as TLC's *A Baby Story,* which follows couples through their final weeks of pregnancy and first days with a newborn, to sitcoms and dramas such as *Modern Family* and *Parenthood,* ensemble narratives portraying family life as inevitable, the source of all the driving emotional arcs for the characters. The social-consumerist site Pinterest offers countless decorating suggestions for parties celebrating procreation: not only baby showers but also gender-reveal gatherings and a kind of elaborate, meet-the-baby party called a Sip and See. Celebrity culture has been particularly fixated on pregnancy, with paparazzi following female stars through their reproductive years, watching for signs of pregnancy like dogged field scientists.

Despite my years of practice and longing, I have always been repelled by pronatal pressure and messaging, which appears to negate the importance of the individual and what she might accomplish aside from breeding. A friend once told me that she didn't like driving a mutual friend, who was pregnant at the time—she didn't want to be responsible, she explained, in case there was an accident. I was in my friend's passenger seat when she admitted this. "But what about me?" I asked, offended that I was less valuable somehow than our other friend's fetus.

I once told this same friend, childless and a decade older than me, that I wanted to have both of my children by the time I was thirty. I was twenty-two, twenty-three. I didn't know anything. The things that I knew were built-in things: models of how to live absorbed and inherited from my mother and from her mother; biologically driven emotions that surfaced when I fell in love, when I held an infant or read to a child. I don't know if this makes them more or less real.

I didn't recover from my baby fever, but I believe that I would have, eventually. I would have fulfilled my longings by caring for the children of others; I would have enjoyed independence, freedom, and time. Instead Richard and I returned to fertility treatment and took what to us were extraordinary measures, finally conceiving our daughter through in vitro fertilization. It is the best decision we've ever made, though of course this appraisal is filtered through the experience of success.

Five years before we started IVF, when Richard and I decided we were ready to start a family, I thought it would be a good time to mention our plans to my gynecologist. I went in for my annual exam and thought about how I should say it, if at all, and whether there was some question I should ask about my health.

I didn't want to say that we were ready to start "trying," which sounded exhibitionist to me. I was always on my best behavior with doctors, proudly (sometimes inaccurately) checking "Never" for smoking and "Less than one alcoholic beverage per day" for drinking and "3–5 times per week" for exercising, and I remember awkwardly waiting, all through the exam, for a good time to bring it up. Finally she asked if I had any questions, and I blurted that I didn't want to take birth control pills anymore, that I planned to get pregnant. It sounded formal and false, like a statement about the future in a job interview. She said something reassuring and positive, but I remember feeling embarrassed and already afraid that things would not go easily.

And they didn't. They don't, for many of us, and we're left with choices: to treat infertility, to have a child alone or with a partner, to adopt domestically or from overseas, to live a childless or child-free life. I became interested in the stories of other people who faced and made these choices, and in the stories that looked different from the ones I'd always been told.

I became interested in the stories that don't get told, the ones some people don't want to hear. I became interested in trying.

Imaginary Children

...

It was ten o'clock on a Tuesday morning in December, and I was waiting to see a matinee performance of that holiday classic, *Who's Afraid of Virginia Woolf?,* with twelve of my AP English students. The drama teacher sat next to me; our kids were one row in front of us. From where we sat, on steep risers, we could see the tops of their heads as they leaned together to talk.

I'd taught at a small, rural charter school for three years; when I started there were barely ten students in most of my classes. Our principal warned us against getting too involved in their lives, but the very structure of the school made it tempting to feel as if the students were our own children—we drove them on field trips in our cars, ate lunch with them, counseled them about boyfriends, girlfriends, problems at home. The same principal, in years past, prepared Thanksgiving dinner for the whole school and their families. The students had our cell phone numbers; they knew where we lived and called some of us by our first names. They could get emotional, fighting with us over grades, attendance, wardrobe choices. Once a student called me a bitch for criticizing a project he was proud of; I sent him out of the room, and he cried for an hour, truly remorseful, in the guidance counselor's office. We knew the things that motivated or upset them, and if they imagined that their teachers talked about them when we gathered for casual chats, they were right. Like parents, we constantly strategized about how to strike the correct balance between what they wanted and what they needed. As we waited for the performance to begin, I worried about an earnest, religious girl who last year recused herself from several reading assignments because of instances of sex or strong language (when we read *Huck Finn,* another student helpfully blacked out the offending words in her copy of the book). I wondered if she'd walk out on this performance, what I'd say when I followed her.

I have loved this play since I first read it as a sophomore in college, though it means something different to me now. Back then, it was about the shock of George and Martha's dysfunction— *You make me puke*—and how they made their way back, after all the fighting, the rounds of "get the guest," to something approaching love. I suspected that that was what interested my students—the verbal histrionics, the cruelty—but they must have also recognized, from the literature we'd read together, a familiar idea within this story of a childless, miserable couple: failing to have children has a socially distorting, morally corrosive effect on people's lives, especially on the lives of women. Three years into my own experience with infertility, I could admit that I once saw this play through the same lens. Now I was attuned to another part of the narrative: the missing child and what George and Martha do to survive his absence.

A couple of months earlier, I left these same students to drive twenty miles to the hospital in Chapel Hill where I'd been receiving fertility treatments for almost a year. No one knew where I was going, only that I'd be back by lunchtime. I remember feeling hopeful and excited in the clear, crisp light of early fall, a time of year that reminds me always of childhood and fresh starts. This was to be my fourth intrauterine insemination, or IUI; after days of testing my urine in the school bathroom using an ovulation-predictor kit, I'd finally achieved the digital smiley face that indicated I was about to ovulate, and I made my appointment.

Richard had already been to the hospital, early that morning, to provide his sample of sperm, which would be washed in a special machine that left only the most capable swimmers. Our chances for conception were slim, but the procedure was relatively affordable and easy to manage. Both financially and in terms of time, scheduling an IUI was like getting a new set of tires—even if sometimes every month; in vitro fertilization, our next step, would be like buying a new car, or several new cars. No one I knew had attempted IUIs expecting them to work the first, or even the second, time; because clinics are not required by the Society for Assisted Reproductive Technologies to keep data on IUI success rates, all we had to go on were the stories of cumulative success or failure shared on message boards or in our support group. Three failed attempts were nothing—I knew women who had been successful after five, six, or seven IUIs. Eventually, I hoped, we'd be successful too.

When the doctor led me not into the dim room with the familiar examination table and stirrups but into a separate, brightly lit conference room, I knew that my hope had been foolish. I hardly looked at the numbers he circled on my chart as he explained the futility of trying the procedure again.

"I think it's time," he said, "to move on to something else."

I knew we weren't ready—financially, emotionally—for IVF. For now, we were done. I took a handful of tissues and drove back to school. It was lunchtime, warm enough for the students to eat outside. I walked to my room without speaking to anyone, closed the door, and locked it. I don't remember if anyone tried to come in, but I do know that none of my high school students ever asked me why I didn't have any children. Perhaps they thought they were enough.

It did not occur to me, when I first read Edward Albee's play, to wonder why George and Martha could not have children. I was nineteen years old, and the mechanics of reproduction had little meaning in my life aside from the birth control pills I took daily. I suppose I realized that Martha, in her early fifties, was beyond her fertile years, but that fact is never discussed directly. In act 3, when their childlessness is laid bare to their guests, Nick and Honey, George and Martha express themselves with uncharacteristic reserve. Nick asks George, quietly, "You couldn't have . . . any?" "*We* couldn't," says George. "*We* couldn't," Martha echoes, with "a hint of communion," according to the stage directions.

George and Martha are past the crisis point of infertility—childbirth is a ship that long ago sailed—and we are not invited to wonder why they did not have children or what they might have done to treat their condition. Instead, the couple represents an idea about what the rest of a childless marriage looks like—the subversion of the traditional heterosexual relationship, the one that progresses, as the school-yard chant goes, from kissing to love to marriage to baby carriage. They are a dangerous couple because they lack the anchoring effect of family. They are inappropriate, vitriolic, unfaithful, lewd, alcoholic. They are thwarted—George in his career, Martha in the expectations she had for George's career—and in their unhappiness, they bring out the worst in their guests. They "get the guest" because they are so unanchored.

"Who's afraid of Virginia Woolf," George sings near the end of the second act. Honey joins him.

"STOP IT!" screams Martha.

Honey leaves the room to vomit.

The house lights came up at intermission, and our students turned to us, blinking and smiling, a little exhausted. Though the actors in this university production lacked a certain sex appeal—Martha was too thin and angular, and George was short, bald, and narrow shouldered—I could tell our kids were enjoying the production. They laughed when George mocked Nick; they gasped when Martha came on to him. I was too busy monitoring their responses to pay much attention to my own. *You okay?* I mouthed to my wary student. She nodded, then left with a friend for the concession booth.

Literature often asks us to imagine the way childlessness affects its protagonists. By the time my AP English class got to George and Martha, they had already read several accounts of childless women and couples, each of them reinforcing this unanchored, subversive quality. Though we had no textbooks, I chose their readings based on suggestions from our state curriculum, availability of opportunities (such as the chance to see a production), and my sense of what these students—these stand-in children—would like. It was a selfish move, though, at its core; I wanted to see the students claim the characters I loved so much as their own, but I also wanted to be the teacher who introduced them. I was thrilled when a girl who did not always do her reading sauntered into class one morning, gleefully impersonating Dickens's shriveled, rejected-at-the-altar Miss Havisham, cruelly exhorting her stand-in daughter, Estella, to break Pip's heart.

And we talked for days about Lady Macbeth, another appealing villain. The Macbeths are presumably not past their child-bearing years, and they imagine the children they might have with a kind of perverse and violent pillow talk. Lady Macbeth tells her husband that if they did have a child and he asked her to kill it, she'd "have pluck'd [her] nipple from his boneless gums" and dashed its brains out. Macbeth responds by fondly telling her she should "bring forth men-children only." They are childless all the same, and plagued by it, surrounded as they are by happier, more virtuous families. Macbeth, heirless, sees Banquo's line of kingly succession as an affront to his own happiness and success. And what does he get up to, spurred by his own ambition and the goading of his childless wife? Murder of Duncan, murder of Banquo, murder of Macduff's whole family—all his "pretty ones." As with George and Martha, as with the brooding Miss Havisham, what the Macbeths lack makes them dangerous.

Sitting in the darkened theater, considering my own state of childlessness, it occurred to me how many of the female characters we talked about most—Hester Prynne, Miss Havisham, Sethe—are defined by their relationship to children, a subtle reinforcement, for my students, that they were at the center of someone else's very identity. In reality, this was both true and not true; some had doting parents, while others had parents who'd disappeared into work, addiction, or other relationships. Still, even the most neglected could not seem to imagine a life that didn't involve parenthood as a milestone. At seventeen or eighteen years old, they already knew the number of children they would like to have and the age they'd like to be when they had them, and most of their plans replicated the family structures they were born into. Those with one sibling thought they'd like to have two children, while those from large families imagined the same for themselves. Even the most romantically inexperienced among them were certain that they would one day have a family.

When Richard and I first lived together, in Los Angeles, we had a collection of small stuffed animals that began with a scarf-wearing bear who came, inexplicably, with my engagement ring. To keep the bear company we added a toy panda, two stuffed hamsters, and a rabbit dressed in pirate costume, and we invented personalities for each of them, bringing them out on holidays for family-style celebrations. We made them tacos on Cinco de Mayo and bought them lottery tickets for Christmas, and we never felt strange about it—it was just something we did—though we never told anyone either.

By now we were painfully aware of the way our rituals and traditions might appear to other people, continuously reminded that our life together did not resemble the lives of our parents at this age, or those of any of our aunts, uncles, or cousins. In-creasingly, our life was less and less like the lives of our mar-ried friends, who had entered a new and somewhat exclusive world of playdates and birthday parties and bedtimes. But our life did not resemble our single or childless friends' lives either. We lived in a constant state of waiting: for the next cycle, the next appointment, the next support-group meeting. We didn't travel far; we saved and saved. We calculated—if this treatment is successful, we will be this far along in June, this far in August.

Sometimes I caught us talking about our imaginary chil-dren. It's not something we did before we started trying, or even before we started failing. We didn't have a list of baby names; we never mentioned children or trying to other people. But some-times I found myself saying "What if she . . ." or "What if he . . ." How old would she have to be to kayak with us? How much would it cost to build a skate ramp in the woods? Then I'd get my period—it always arrived, if not exactly like clockwork—and we were back to where we started.

We count on literature to prepare us, to console us, but I am shocked by how little consolation there is for the infertile, or even for those who are childless by choice and trying to live in a world that is largely fertile and family driven. Old ideas and prejudices persist—a woman without a child is less feminine, less nurturing. She is defined by what she does not have, and she confronts, again and again, a culture that reinforces the wrongness of her circumstances, which may be biological or social, temporary or permanent, something she treats or some-thing she accepts.

For the infertile-but-trying woman, even the way she chooses to treat her condition is subject to literary commentary, literary example. Think of the biblical Sarah, barren to the age of ninety, who endured and even blessed Abraham's procreation with the maid before God finally gave her a child. The allegorical message of her story is that by accepting God's will with patience and faith, Sarah was rewarded with the birth of Isaac long after it should have been biologically possible. Though Abraham's wife had little other choice than to wait, the act of waiting transformed her—from Sarai to Sarah, from childless and grieving to the mother of nations.

The myth of Sarah infects our literature and our thinking, and it offers insight into what makes the spectacle of Albee's Martha, who responds to her childlessness by inventing a son, so pitiable and grotesque. Conception is transformative but also mysterious, endowed by God rather than planned by the woman. To interfere is to be unnatural, greedy, grasping.

Looking back on my first book of short stories, I see how thoroughly the myth was part of my own thinking. I did not anticipate trouble becoming pregnant when I wrote the stories, but motherhood, that long-expected stage of life, must have been on my mind. I included three characters who happen to be infertile and one character who is accidentally pregnant.

It's interesting to me now how thoroughly those characters replicate received wisdom about fertility. Loretta is a nurse who is saving for a boat, the *Mattaponi Queen,* to enjoy in her retirement. Though she and her late husband had no children, she accepts her infertility stoically. Accompanying her elderly patient, Cutie, to the Dairy Queen, she remembers going out for soft serve with her husband on Friday nights: "We would sit on the cement benches and eat our cones like a dating couple, never mentioning that it would have been more fun if we had children with us." Though a few readers have told me that they find Loretta prickly or dishonest, she is as close to a hero as the collection has, and the stories in which she appears honor the way she accepts her condition, mourns it privately, and focuses her energy on other kinds of caretaking. Of course, there is nothing wrong with Loretta's acceptance and privacy, or with finding her emotional strength and resourcefulness admirable.

My portrayal of her nonmedicalized endurance becomes problematic for me in the context of a minor character who appears in another of my stories.

Jessica is the infertile daughter of Melinda, whose husband, Jonas, is in the process of gender reassignment. Writing the story, I worried a lot about portraying Jonas's and Melinda's experiences accurately; I did research about middle-aged couples like them and about the hormone therapy and surgeries in Jonas's future. In contrast, I hardly remember researching Jessica's condition and treatment at all. I suppose I thought I knew enough.

Jessica is only twenty-two; while not impossible, it's rare for someone her age to be infertile. She takes fertility pills for six months, then has a "half-dozen fertilized eggs . . . implanted in her womb" and—in Melinda's words—"lies on her side all day and gives herself injections in the butt." I'm not sure how I came up with this course of treatment, but I now know it to be inaccurate. More damning is my portrayal of Jessica; she is narrow minded, desperate, and emotionally unavailable to her family, and her pursuit of infertility treatment is directly linked to these characteristics. "Stress is the enemy of conception," she warns her mother before hanging up on her, right after Melinda delivers the news about Jonas's sex change. The treatment has not only isolated her but has also made her less attractive and feminine in the eyes of Melinda, who laments to her sister that Jessica "wears sweatpants to the grocery story and goes out without her hair done."

If Loretta is like the biblical Sarah, patient and accepting and stoic, then Jessica represents a newer stereotype that has accompanied medically sophisticated infertility treatment: the desperate, uptight woman who blindly pursues conception at all costs, destroying her relationships and her dignity in the process. If I could go back and rewrite her, I would. Though I'd still want her character to provide a contrast to her open-minded mother, I would not choose to make IVF the means of

expressing Jessica's selfishness. At the very least, I would get
the details of her treatment right.

Why didn't I concern myself with portraying Jessica's treatment
accurately? I suppose the answer may be because popular culture has provided us with so many consistent portrayals of the
IVF patient—needy, self-focused, materialistic, unnatural—that
I assumed they must be accurate. But I think that there is an
even more compelling, and more troubling, reason that connects back to George and Martha, back to the Macbeths, and
back to Sarah.

As a culture, we in the Western world have imagined human
conception as mysterious, even magical. We can hope or pray
for a child, but it is nature or God who will ultimately decide
whether that child is conceived and born. This way of thinking has a positive social effect; it makes mothers and fathers
feel chosen and special, and may help soothe the burden of un-
planned or unwanted pregnancies. But think about the infertile
couple: despite their prayers, hopes, or wishes, they have not
been selected by God or nature to have a child. There is something wrong with them—biologically, maybe morally. They
are broken, unsuitable for parenting. Perhaps their love is not
strong enough, or perhaps they want different things. Perhaps
they are too concerned with witchcraft and regicide, like the
Macbeths. Maybe they are too old, like George and Martha.
Maybe they fight too much.

And if they choose to intervene, are they defying God? Defying nature? In 1962, the year that *Who's Afraid of Virginia
Woolf?* premiered, scientists were still more than a decade away
from the first successful in vitro fertilization treatment, yet the
specter of the test-tube baby is present in George's debates with
Nick. "You people are going to make them in test tubes, aren't
you? You biologists," George accuses. More recently, Catholic
teaching, which regularly addresses questions of bioethics and

medicine, has opposed many forms of assisted reproduction, including IVF, staunchly and consistently. The wide-ranging objections raised by Catholic bishops and bioethicists to IVF include the creation and destruction of unviable or unwanted embryos; the genetic screening and selection of embryos; the profiteering of doctors; the use of donor eggs or sperm; the temptation of human cloning; and the idea that it is all too technical and artificial. Even Jesus, according to the Nicene Creed, was "begotten, not made." The root objection, however, appears to be the way that assisted reproduction interferes with natural conception, which is seen as a gift from God. In 1987, Pope John Paul II issued the *Donum Vitae* (full title: *Instruction on Respect for Human Life in Its Origin and on the Dignity of Procreation*), which asserted that IVF deprived procreation "of its proper perfection." In 2012 Pope Benedict XVI, who cowrote the *Donum Vitae,* expanded on this idea in an address to two hundred scientists and members of the Pontifical Academy for Life at a conference on "the diagnosis and treatment of infertility." He likened IVF treatment to "taking the Creator's place" and encouraged infertile couples to "find a response that fully respects their dignity as persons and spouses."

I am not Catholic, or even religious, but I notice that my state-provided health insurance coverage for infertility matches the recommendations in the *Donum Vitae:* hormonal and surgical treatment of my body is okay, but "any means of attempting pregnancy that does not involve normal coitus" is not. Further, before experiencing infertility myself, I can see that I had somehow taken on this bias against assisted reproduction, which is in itself a bias against the many infertile couples who have sought treatment. It is more comforting to imagine a baby who arrives (for free!) via chance or grace or biology than one who is created, at great (and for many, prohibitive) expense, in a sterile laboratory. And it is true that many of the rituals and practices of assisted reproduction lack dignity; they are not what I imagined, anyway, when I thought about having children. It is undignified to inject yourself with hormones designed to slow or enhance ovarian production. It is undignified to have your ovaries monitored by transvaginal ultrasound; to be sedated so that your eggs can be aspirated into a needle; to have your husband emerge sheepishly from a locked room with the "sample" that will be combined with your eggs under supervision of an embryologist. The grainy photo they hand you on transfer day, of your eight-celled embryo (which does not look remotely like a baby), is undignified, and so is all the waiting and despairing that follows.

But many things in life, and especially in marriage and medicine, are undignified. One could argue that certain diets lack dignity, as do going to the gym, having a colonoscopy, and performing many kinds of home repair. And when was sex ever dignified? I don't think that when the former pope advised couples to find a more respectful response to infertility, he was concerned about a woman's feet in stirrups or her eggs in a dish. I think the real trouble is with her unfulfilled desire—her grasping, her wanting, her circumventing. It's the idea that she is so dissatisfied with how things are that she would turn to elective medicine (as I have) or to the imagination (as Martha did). Better to wait, like Sarah (mother of Isaac), like Hannah (mother of the prophet Samuel), like Elizabeth (mother of John the Baptist).

Resistance to the things that are, particularly resistance that fails, is undignified. One of the things I love about Albee's play is the gradual way it allows us to discern, within Martha's rawness and apparent lack of control, an essential gravity and fortitude. When she admiringly characterizes Nick's study of biology as "less . . . abstruse" than that of mathematics, George corrects her—"Abstract"—and she fires back "ABSTRUSE! In the sense of recondite," then sticks out her tongue. She is dignified on her own terms, and it is up to the audience to catch up to her.

Initially, some playgoers and critics struggled with the details of George and Martha's marriage, and with Martha's character particularly. The first review heard by Albee and some members of the cast, received and transcribed via telephone, was from Robert Coleman of the *Daily Mirror,* who wrote, "This is a sick play about sick people. They are neurotic, cruel and nasty. They really belong in a sanitarium for the mentally ill rather than on the stage." The play was recommended, in a *New York Daily News* headline, FOR DIRTY-MINDED FEMALES ONLY (which served only to increase ticket sales); later, calling the play "filthy" and rejecting its unanimous selection by the award committee, the 1963 Pulitzer advisory board refused to award a prize for theater. Aside from the profanity and the vociferous, unabated arguing of George and Martha, many were troubled in particular by the presence of the imaginary son. Some argued that George and Martha represented a homosexual relationship in disguise (Albee, who is gay, rejected this idea); Richard Schechner, writing for the *Tulane Drama Review,* asserted that the "illusory child" was "neither philosophically, psychologically, nor poetically valid."

This debate over the validity of the imaginary child threatened the film version of *Who's Afraid of Virginia Woolf?* too. Ernest Lehman, the producer and screenwriter, proposed dealing with critical discomfort by making George and Martha's imaginary son real. In Lehman's suggested version, Jim would have hung himself in a closet at the age of sixteen. The wallpapered-over closet would have served as a crass physical representation of the question of "truth or illusion" that George and Martha spar over throughout the play.

Albee, who was adopted as an infant by wealthy parents he later described as emotionally distant, had some reason to think about infertility and its consequences. "The whole family was barren: the end of the line," he has said of the Albee clan. "Skidding to an awful halt. The whole lot of them." (His father's sister was also infertile.) Albee knew of his adoption from an early age, and he experienced his role in the family as somewhat imaginary—that is, he was meant to fill a particular role. "They bought me," he said of his parents. "They paid $133.30." It's not difficult to imagine that Albee might sympathize with George and Martha as well as "sonny-Jim," the child who does not exist, and it must have felt strange to him, the same way it does to me now, to hear a central element of his play dismissed as unrealistic or, worse, invalid.

Before the play was produced, Albee wrote to Leonard Woolf to let him know that his late wife's name would appear in the title. Woolf wrote back with his approval, and after seeing it performed in London wrote back again, asking if Albee had read one of Virginia Woolf's stories, "Lappin and Lapinova." "The details are quite different but the theme is the same as that of the imaginary child in your play," Woolf told him. The story is about a newly married couple, Ernest and Rosalind, who cope with the pressures of married life by inventing, as the story puts it, "a private world, inhabited, save for the one white hare, entirely by rabbits." As Lappin and Lapinova, the king and queen of their imagined world, they are able to feel connected in the face of an alternately dull and threatening reality. Like George and Martha, they agree to tell no one: "That was the point of it; nobody save themselves knew that such a world existed." But the strongest connection between Albee's play and Woolf's story (which Albee said he had not read) is the destruction of the imaginary world, which is also accomplished by the husband. Lapinova has been "caught in a trap," he tells Rosalind, "killed." Rosalind is no longer allowed to live in a fantasy world, and their marriage (unlike, we presume, George and Martha's) is destroyed.

In *Infertility and the Creative Spirit,* Roxane Head Dinkin and Robert J. Dinkin write that "envisioning a fantasy child is not as unusual as one might think, and fantasy children appear not only in fictional works but in the lives of actual people." Among the writers they identify who actively imagined children are Ella Wheeler Wilcox, who invented, with her husband, the life of a daughter named Winifred; Katherine Mansfield, who fantasized with her husband about a boy named Dicky; and Dr. Seuss, who with his wife Helen had an imaginary child named Chrysanthemum-Pearl.

The stuffed-animal family Richard and I collected in Los Angeles lived in our bedroom, as if in a dollhouse, on a shelf made to hold CDs. Eleven years later, in North Carolina, I put the bear, the panda, the rabbit, and the hamsters in a basket, along with their losing lottery tickets and old Christmas candy, and shoved the whole thing under the bed. Sometimes Richard would mention them—"We haven't seen them for a while"—and I'd make excuses about the lack of space, my aversion to clutter. In truth, I didn't want to think about the way our peculiar habit would look to outsiders, or contemplate the possibility that we'd still be making tacos for stuffed animals while our friends went to school plays and graduations. Around this time our support group had grown, and a number of women were in active ART cycles. No one talked about imaginary children; we spent most of our precious two hours discussing more pressing matters, like the benefits of acupuncture and how to inject Follistim with the least amount of discomfort. We had time only for the body, never the imagination.

In the classroom, it had taken a while for my more literal-minded students to understand that George and Martha's bouncing baby boy isn't real. "What?" they said, turning back pages. "He's dead? He's *not* dead? He never existed?" But in the darkened theater, as the devastation of act 3 unfolded before them, they understood; I watched them bracing themselves as George announced, with menacing triumph, "I've got a surprise for you, baby."

George and Martha's son is a product of sorrow and disappointment but also of imagination. They do not have enough to do; they must fill their days and nights somehow, and it's easy for me to imagine how idle talk and speculation about the child they might have had transformed itself into a boy with a name and a twenty-first birthday. He is so real to them that, like some people's actual children, he becomes a weapon. In front of their guests, George insinuates maternal smothering that borders on sexual abuse, while Martha suggests that in fact, he might not even be George's son.

There is sweetness in their imagining, too—when Martha says the boy, away at college, only writes to her, George claims to have a stack of letters from his son, and Martha describes his "easy birth," his "full head of black, fine, fine hair which, oh, later, later, became as blond as the sun." But her most vivid imaginings are the memories she conjures of the woman she might have been—the couple they might have been—had they had the child they wanted. "He walked evenly between us," she remembers, "a hand out to each of us for what we could offer by way of support, affection, teaching, even love." I find the play almost unbearably painful as she recounts the intricately imagined banana boats she made for him on Sundays, "a whole peeled banana, scooped out on top, with green grapes for the crew," and "along the sides, stuck to the boat with toothpicks, orange slices . . . SHIELDS."

Here's one question the play provokes: are George and Martha the way they are because they could not have children, or are they denied children because of the way they are? It is a chicken-and-egg dilemma that goes back to the Macbeths, back to Sarah, back to the insensitive comments every infertile couple dreads.

And here is another: how are we to read George's killing of their son with the made-up telegram, before their stricken guests? If we read their son as a symbol of what is wrong in George and Martha's relationship, of lies and deception and the refusal to see things for how they are, the killing is an act of mercy. That's how I read the play, years and years ago, and it's how most of my students read it too.

"Who's afraid of Virginia Woolf . . . ," George sings softly.

"I . . . am . . . George," says Martha. "I . . . am."

The houselights came up. The drama teacher and I quickly wiped away tears.

"He had to do it," our students said on the way back to school. "He had to do it so they could face reality, so there could be some hope left in their marriage."

"Is there hope?" I asked. "Do you think tomorrow will be good for them?"

"Maybe not good," they demurred. "Better?"

Instinctively, my students understood Martha's creation of an imaginary son as transgressive, intuiting the same cultural logic that former pope Benedict relied on when he dismissed IVF as beneath human dignity. Her creation of the boy is a refusal to accept things as they are. What my students didn't understand, because they were so young, is that there are many ways to live in a marriage, and many things you must do to survive a long one. What if Jim is necessary? What if his green eyes and those banana boats are all that Martha and George have that is good? What if by killing Jim, George is killing something vital?

That's the way Richard reads George's killing of Jim—as violence, as cruelty. It's for this reason that he finds the play painful and difficult to read. The life of the imagination is more important to him than the destruction of illusions.

I agree with him, though I don't believe Albee would. Act 3 is, after all, called "The Exorcism," and Albee has carefully woven in admissions from Martha that there is more to sustain their marriage than cruelty and games: "There is only one man in my life who has ever . . . made me happy," she tells the disbelieving Nick.

But then, what do you do with the play's title, with the ghost of Virginia Woolf? I made a note to tell my students more about her: that she was brilliant, that she influenced generations of writers. I could tell them I first read her when I was their age; maybe we had time to read *To the Lighthouse* or *Mrs. Dalloway.* Maybe they already knew some things about her: that she was married and had no children, that she suffered from mental illness, that she walked into the River Ouse with heavy stones in her pocket and drowned.

(Who's afraid of Virginia Woolf?)

(I am.)

For Halloween that year, I dressed for school as Miss Havisham, wearing a yellowed, lacy debutante dress and carrying a plate of spiderwebbed cake and a deck of playing cards. "Break their hearts!" I hissed at my students from beneath my veil. Most of the other teachers dressed up for Halloween too, and our choices usually revealed something about our subjects or how we perceived ourselves—the outdoor education teacher came to school as a "canoe accident," covered in fake blood and bruises; the vain and handsome Latin teacher came as Superman. The year before, I was Lady Macbeth, binding my hair, coating my hands with red, and sleepwalking through the halls.

Our participation in what is essentially a childhood ritual— dressing up, pretending—delighted the students, who saw us as extensions of their families. They wanted to carpool with us and camp with us and watch episodes of *Doctor Who* with us at evening lock-ins. They wanted us taking pictures at their dances and proms. They asked to be our Facebook friends. I had students, frustrated by the reasonable or unreasonable actions of their real parents, beg me to adopt them.

I don't remember looking for the same kind of access to my teachers when I was their age, but I have always been close to my students, baking for them, inviting them to museums and plays. My classroom's family atmosphere is my creation and an expression of my need, too. I know that the stories I put in front of them—and, to a lesser degree, that the stories I write—matter. They are patterns not only for how to live, but also for how to see the world. For all the variety, beauty, and brilliance of the works read in a typical high school English class, though, there is a sameness to their treatment of reproduction and reproductive choices. Maybe that sameness reflects a need to understand ourselves within the contexts of our families—we are each of us (even Macduff) born to someone—but what happens when one of them, like me, cannot have a child? What if she needs medical intervention to conceive? What if she chooses not to? What will she read then?

On Halloween, we offered the students extra credit for dressing in historical or literary costumes, and some of them annoyed me (on purpose, I believe) by dressing as characters from *Harry Potter* or *Twilight*. But this year, one girl wore a long gown in a printed African cotton and painted a birthmark in the shape of a stemmed rose around her eye. I knew right away that she was Toni Morrison's Sula, who embraces a more openly unconventional life—sexually liberated, without a husband or children or a permanent home—than any of my students had ever admitted considering for herself.

"I'm Sula, fool," she said when one of her classmates asked about her costume. Then, more kindly: "I love her."

My students nodded; eventually, they had all loved *Sula*. But we struggled with that book at first. Morrison's deeply imbedded authorial perspective, her lack of exposition, her very casualness—about sex, about drugs and death and mental illness and racism—challenged them. I'd finally broken through by sitting on the edge of a desk, as I used to when I taught younger students, and reading whole chapters aloud while they sat with their heads resting on their arms, like schoolchildren. Like my children.

In the Peanut Hospital

• • •

My mother wouldn't tell me the name of her surgery—it was for old ladies, and she didn't want to talk about it. No, it wasn't dangerous, yes, she'd stay the night in a hospital, and she wanted me there and at home with her for a few days afterward. My father would be there too, but he wasn't good around sick people or hospitals, though he'd been a sick person in a hospital twice in recent memory.

I'm not sick, she assured me. There's nothing *wrong* with me. It's a female surgery, she said, like that answered things.

I made plans to drive to Virginia, to the distant hospital in Suffolk where her doctor practiced. We had reservations at a Quality Inn that looked seedy even on the website (unlike the spiffier Holiday Inn Express, the Quality Inn would allow my parents' dog).

It was August of the hottest year on record. Along the highway, grasses and weeds were yellowed and burnt. Out west, farmers struggled to feed their livestock; hay was high, water dear. A drought map of North Carolina showed every county in dangerous red-brown territory, and our well at home had to be managed carefully: brief showers, short laundry cycles, no guests. The Haw River was drained to a bathwater stillness, too low to paddle more than short stretches.

What bothers me, a biologist friend told me the last time we were on the water together, *is the idea that there is something wrong with me. The idea that I am damaged, faulty.*

She was strong, healthy, beautiful, successful. She was also infertile. Our shared condition was why we met, through another friend who knew about our mutual struggle. Of course, I told her, you aren't damaged. But her body wasn't working the way she wanted it to, and mine wasn't either.

What is wrong with having something wrong with you, I wondered on my drive to Virginia—windows closed, too hot then for anything but the blaring air conditioner. I had told my mother almost as little about my infertility or treatment as she had now told me about her surgery. Our broken parts—the broken female parts, at least—were an uncommon silence between us.

In *Of Woman Born,* her book of memoir and cultural criticism about the patriarchy-suffused experience of motherhood, Adrienne Rich writes about the need women felt in her youth to present to the world an image of health, industry, and fertility. Already a serious poet when she married at twenty-four, she remembers taking up a broom the day after her wedding, thinking, *"This is what women have always done."* While Rich was ambivalent about how motherhood would affect her ambitions (by the birth of her first child, she'd won the Yale Younger Poets prize, and before her marriage she had wanted to travel and become a journalist), she knew that "to have a child was to assume adult womanhood to the full, to prove myself, to be 'like other women.'" As a pregnant woman—she had three sons in quick succession—she writes that she felt, "for the first time in my adolescent and adult life, not-guilty. The atmosphere of approval in which I was bathed—even by strangers on the street, it seemed—was like an aura I carried with me, in which doubts, fears, misgivings, met with absolute denial."

The pregnant body suggests a story we think we know: health, love, happiness. That pregnancy is in fact a dangerous condition that tends to make women poorer and more vulnerable to violence and some diseases—and certainly less likely to write books—isn't something we talk about. We instead learn, early on, that the inconveniences particular to the female body—getting a period, wearing a bra, worrying about becoming or not becoming pregnant—are properly suffered in secret, even in shame. We learn not to talk about "doubts, fears, misgivings," related to the female body—and we celebrate instead the visible condition of pregnancy, in part because it is so visually obvious but also because it has been done *to* a woman and can be seen (incorrectly) as something she endures or even passively enjoys rather than as something she has to handle.

My own mother remembers her 1970s pregnancies with a fondness that emphasizes how natural and intuitive they were. She didn't have an ultrasound for either pregnancy but "knew" that I was a girl and my brother was a boy. In fact, she didn't see a doctor—there were no obstetricians in our county—until she was seven months along with me, and he and my mother disagreed about my due date (she was right, the doctor almost a month off). Both of her births were natural births. That was the story she told me.

Except, I learned later, for the Demerol she took intravenously in the last stage of labor with me. Of course I wouldn't have judged my mom for any pain relief she needed, opiates or an epidural or even complete sedation, which Rich experienced for all three of her births. But my mother needed the story of my birth to be about nature taking its course and the perfection of the experience. "You didn't even cry," she always told me proudly.

Blond, five feet tall, and one hundred pounds, my mother sits on a pillow to see over the steering wheel of her fourteen-year-old Mercedes station wagon and was once pulled over by a county sheriff who assumed she was a child on a joyride. On school field trips, as parent chaperone, she was often mistaken for a student by my teachers and was once yanked up by her hair while she tried to get something out of our lunch bag (that this would be considered an appropriate thing to do to a child is another matter). Her lifestyle is a specialized one: she knows how to build a roaring fire in a woodstove but not where the gas goes in her car. I've registered several email accounts for her, but she has never checked them, not once. For a small person, she has large bones—big, knobby artist's hands, knock-knees. Her shoes (she has many; none are sneakers) are boats. Scoliosis, uncorrected in her childhood, makes her short-torsoed, and her arms and legs are disproportionately long and thin. She excels at rowing, kayaking, and waterskiing and walks like a New Yorker with somewhere to be; I have never seen her run or play a team sport.

Before my grandmother died, it was a tradition in my family for the women (my grandmother, my mother, and my aunt) to attend their yearly mammograms together, on the same day. Maybe you can credit the pervasive pink-ribbon campaigns, but breast health appeared to exist in a separate realm from other women's health issues—not a source of embarrassment but a chance for bonding. On mammogram day my mother, aunt, and grandmother each took their turn at the imaging machine and then went out for lunch and pedicures. Once, when I was in college, Mom had a follow-up appointment at a specialist's office near my apartment in Richmond. I met her there to wait with her, and while she was gone—it felt like hours—I had a panic attack in the floral-wallpapered waiting room. I felt suddenly as though a lobe of my left lung had slipped through my rib cage and was caught on one of the bones. I couldn't sit up in my chair and had to lean over, breathing shallowly, until she returned. Just a problem with the machine, she explained lightly. It took my breathing and posture the rest of the day to recover.

Before I had a child, whenever I imagined what was most

terrifying to me, it was always the loss of my mother. Ostrich-like, I tried to avoid it, like thoughts of climate change, water shortages: inevitable catastrophes, a long way off. It was the "greatest disaster that could happen," as Virginia Woolf remembered the death of her own beloved mother. William Maxwell, another writer who lost his mother young, fictionalized mother loss in *So Long, See You Tomorrow* similarly as "the worst that could happen."

"After that," he wrote, "there were no more disasters." Maxwell was writing from the perspective of a lonely, abandoned boy, recounting the immediate atmosphere of shocked, uncommunicative despair that overtook his household. Woolf writes about her mother's death directly, as an abandonment that happened and continued to happen, until her own life (shorter than her mother's short one) ended.

Childlessness bound me to my mother in a strange way—at my age she had two children and was busy making school lunches and dinners, overseeing after-school activities, keeping the house running. She talked to her mother regularly but not every day, as I did (there was no telephone for a while on the farm where we lived when I was little, and then only a party line).

Other than Richard, she was the person I knew best, the person I imagined there with me for all the biggest moments of my life. She accompanied me on parts of my first book tour, fetching coffee for us in the mornings but also losing her wallet (stuffed with cash earned selling flowers at the Walkerton Farmers' Market) along the way. She expertly read subway maps but nearly fainted when she stepped in gum. I found the wallet, iced her sandaled foot and peeled away the gum. She took care of me, and I took care of her.

I suppose what I was most afraid of, when I thought of losing her, was an untethering from family, from female-kind. Who would wait with me in a few years while I took my turn at the mammogram machine? My brother called us "the non-kid-having cousins" because all of our adult cousins had children, while we, in our way, *were* children: still reporting our achievements to our parents, eager for their approval. We had no non-kid-having models in our family—our surfer uncle had a son, and his son had two kids. Our unstable aunt? Two kids, still in college, or so we were told. My dad's two brothers had kids, and their kids had kids—we weren't even sure how many at this point—while *our* parents, for years, talked of granddogs and grandcats.

I waited with Gus, my parents' mini schnauzer and a fine approximation of a toddler, while my mother completed pre-op paperwork in the hospital and my dad paced the parking lot, talking on his cell phone. Mini schnauzers are known for attaching fiercely to one owner, and Gus is heartbroken when my mother leaves him. He splayed at my feet on the hot sidewalk, dejected. Occasionally he thought he recognized a Walkerton neighbor ambling in or out of the hospital's automatic doors and perked up and stood at attention until the stranger passed without admiring him.

She didn't have a good feeling about the hospital, my mother said on her return, bending to take Gus's gently offered paw. It was so far from home, and everyone inside looked sick. Not hospital-sick, she said. Life-sick. Why hadn't she switched doctors already? Her mother was gone, and she barely spoke to my aunt. But here we were: suffering in Suffolk.

The motel had a turbid, greenish swimming pool, and the nonsmoking rooms smelled of smoke. We killed time by carefully checking the beds for bedbugs, scratching imaginary bites, changing into rooms that weren't any better, and walking Gus around the far corners of the property, where we could find the shade and privacy he required to do his business. We were the first party seated at the only sit-down restaurant in town.

The next morning we checked Mom in to the surgical center. She looked smaller than ever on the gurney when we kissed her goodbye. I wasn't worried about the surgery, exactly; I knew it was low risk (though I still didn't know the name or even the goal of the operation) and that she'd spend only a single night in the hospital. My father, by contrast, had recovered for almost a week in a hospital after his triple bypass and even longer for a follow-up surgery that nearly killed him. He'd come away from that experience changed. Sometimes now his feet hurt almost too badly to walk, and he was more prone to the kind of blunt, death-anticipating commentary I associate with the elderly. I suppose that was what I worried about most: that the surgery would change her.

My dad and I took turns walking around the hospital, which had been donated by and named for the Obici family, of the Planters peanut fortune. A Mr. Peanut statue greeted patients in the lobby. The gift shop sold a complement of "Lil' Peanut" baby gifts—onesies, bibs, blankets—though I read, in a commemorative hospital exhibit, that Amedeo and Louise Obici could not have children. The display suggested that they focused instead on charity work, on helping the children in their community.

I thought of two of my friends at home, both going through their first IVF cycles. I would miss our support-group meeting this month, but I imagined using my turn around the table, in September, to tell the story of wandering the peanut hospital while my mom had some unnamed female surgery. This was what I liked best about attending the group—storytelling, recounting the lowest or strangest moments of the month before—though lately it felt as though we had devolved into more practical discussions. Which doctor to consult, which pills to try, which medication to inject where. Maybe we'd evolved instead; maybe the practical was more hopeful—I thought this sometimes, until we returned, next month, and found that the pills and supplements and injections described so earnestly the month before hadn't worked. The narrative failed because it was about only one thing: becoming pregnant. I needed my story to be more flexible.

Mom came out of anesthesia crying. Common, a nurse-anesthesiologist friend told me later: teenage boys fight, and older women cry.

I stood next to her and took her hand. "What's wrong? Are you hurting?"

"I'm crying about my sister," she said bitterly.

"Do you want me to call her?"

"No!"

My mother and her sister had barely spoken for more than a year, since my grandmother's death and an ugly fight over her estate. My aunt wanted to sell my grandmother's things at an estate sale. My mom thought this was tacky and care-less; plus, she wanted everything for herself. Then she found out that my aunt had raided my grandmother's bank account before she died. Now we weren't allowed to say my aunt's name. This was another benefit of having children, I thought—with so many tethers, you could afford to let some go.

The nurse, a smiling, middle-aged woman, checked my mom's vitals but didn't seem concerned about her tears or nausea. She told me that she wished *she* could have the surgery my mom had just had, like maybe my mom was ungrateful, and I wondered again what it was that had been done to her. Nothing glamorous, surely. And why couldn't this woman, a nurse in a hospital, have any surgery she needed?

"It comes from having kids," the nurse told me. "You can't hold your pee."

You can't hold your pee? This was obviously something my mom hadn't wanted me to know, but here was the nurse, talking as if my mother wasn't in the room. I looked over at her, tiny in the hospital bed and writhing in discomfort.

"I think she needs something," I told the nurse. "For nausea."

They all say they need something, the nurse said. *It's normal.*

I held my mom's hand and danced a jig to make her feel better. These were the things I knew how to do: child things, diversions. I reprised our suffering in Suffolk joke and made fun of the nurse, slightly out of her earshot.

"I could stay here," I suggested, patting the guest cot by the window. "It's nicer than the motel."

My dad, returning from his phone-calling peregrinations, thought this was a good idea: he'd go home to Walkerton, get a good night's sleep, and pick us up in the morning. He'd already packed the car. Here was my bag. Have fun, feel better, he loved us.

My parents are progressive, liberal people, but in their forty-plus years together, they've assumed old-fashioned gender roles—my mom does all the cooking, even fried chicken and barbecue (she is vegetarian); my dad fixes the many things that can go wrong in a two-hundred-year-old house. She stayed home with us and painted in spare moments; he worked as a carpenter and contractor. In particular, my mother has done most of the caretaking our family has needed. She took care of my father's mother before she died of cancer, and of his brother, another cancer victim, before that.

Raised for ten years of her life in the nursing home run by her grandmother Donna, she must have picked up on the mix of gentleness and toughness it required, the strong stomach, the unflappability, the constant attention to pills, the clock, and laundry. Donna's patients lived in relative luxury, surrounded by the kinds of things they would have had in their own homes: silver tea services and fine china and pressed linens. The doors to their rooms stood wide open, and my mother, who identified strongly with Kay Thompson's spoiled and neglected Eloise, visited them daily to ask for treats or make silly faces, but she saw, all around her, the constant work of keeping them clean and fed and alive. At night, some of the patients had terrors and would scream or moan until my great-grandmother or another nurse could soothe them. Once, working to resuscitate a dying man, a nurse fainted, and Donna kicked her under the bed and continued chest compressions. She trained her staff to be endlessly polite, mentioning disability or illness with embarrassed euphemisms; incontinent patients were asked if they had to make water.

I have sometimes thought I inherited this gentle-toughness too. In the Brooklyn elementary school where I taught in my twenties, I was the go-to replacement for the squeamish, and I remember cleaning an unfortunate kindergartener, another teacher's student, head to toe after a bathroom accident. The custodian noticed me crouched beside the girl with my rapidly diminishing box of wet wipes and said, approvingly, "You a country girl, Ms. Boggs."

It was one of the best compliments I received in that school and something I remind myself of when I have to deal with unexpected messes. But I was hardly any help at all when my grandmother developed Alzheimer's-type dementia—no good at what we called the bathroom business, when my mother and I visited together and were left to care for Jeannie on our own. Mom did it all—walking her to the toilet, easing her onto the seat, wiping her bottom—while I stood in the doorway, spraying Febreze.

She had her own difficulty with caring for her mother—she could not stand it when Jeannie took out her false teeth (which was often) and would turn away, crying, "No! Put them back in, Mama!" There was something painful and poignant in hearing her call my grandmother Mama, the name she'd used as a child, when Jeannie had so little awareness of our relationships and how we fit together.

Once Jeannie asked, while I was reading to her from *The*

Little Prince, a book she might have read to me, "Where is my mommy?"

"Here I am!" my mother answered. "What do you need?"

There was no regret and no self-pity in identifying herself as her mother's mother, perhaps because she'd been my mother too. This shape-shifting, transforming from child to nurse to parent and back again, is the caretaker's neatest trick, and one that evaded me. I feared becoming only a mother to my mother, a lopsided orbit that would leave me, eventually, alone.

Midafternoon, I decided to take a walk while my mother slept. I wrote my cell phone number on the whiteboard in her room, next to Goals for Today ("Manage nausea," "Walk"). Turning left and following the yellowish corridor, I exited the wing next to an infant's nursery. There were people waiting, grandmas and grandpas, kids, holding pink and blue balloons, flowers and teddy bears. *That one,* a proud father said, pointing at the glass. I didn't look but took out my phone and scrolled to my brother's number.

"Make a casserole or something for after I leave," I bossed him once I got outside. The sun was blazing; there was nowhere shaded to walk, hardly even any grassy spaces. I'd once imagined the birth of my own child—the people who would have waited for us—but now steeled myself to be the one waiting while my brother and his wife were in the delivery room. They weren't expecting, not yet, but I was afraid of the jealousy I imagined for myself. I was already jealous of the capability I assumed they had, and ashamed.

"This is hard," I told him.

"I know," he said. "I'm sorry."

I found a different way back to my mother's room. We tried watching television, got bored, and for a while I amused my mother by reading, from my laptop, a semipublic email rant from a disgraced former editor of a magazine I'd once written for. I shouted the all-caps parts and lowered my voice for the salacious parts about feet. I acted out a drunken come-on and read the goofily profane texts.

"No," she said, clutching her side. "Laughing hurts."

She held my arm on the way to the bathroom but didn't want help changing the diaper-sized pad they'd given her for bleeding; she kept the door closed while she fumbled with it herself. I still had no real idea what they'd done, what stitching or removing or internal adjusting. I hadn't googled it or asked the dismissive nurse for more details. All my mother would say was, "It feels *wrong*." All the doctor would say, on his brief visit earlier, was that everything had gone perfectly.

My mother fell asleep once it was dark outside, and I lay on my side on the narrow, padded bench, covered in as many thin hospital blankets as I could scrounge. I'm good at falling asleep—a farm-kid's talent—but if I wake up, it's hard to find my way back. Sometime after midnight I became aware of noises. They were muffled at first, as if in a dream, then louder as a hall door opened and my mind focused. Someone was moaning in pain; someone else was shushing and soothing. It went on for a while, and I remember being afraid my mother's pain medicine would wear off and she'd soon be moaning too.

I'd imagined that everyone on our quiet wing had been given my mother's still-unnamed surgery or some similar minor corrective. But then I heard the unmistakable cause: a baby crying, shocked and sudden, right next to our room. We weren't near the maternity ward, as I'd assumed walking past the nursery; we were in it, and all around us, all night, women moaned, grunted, and pushed. Their babies—miraculous, tiny, with perfect, messy, mewling cries—were born, wrapped in blankets, handed back to them; were snuggled and breast-fed; had their fingers and toes counted, and counted again. *This is as close as you may ever get,* I thought. It was all so perfectly awful—my aging mother in bed not ten feet away while women labored all around me—that it felt like a message from the universe. *This is as close as you ever* will *get.*

I pulled the blankets over my head, the thin pillow too. By now the sheet I'd stretched over the bench cushions had come untucked, and I pressed my face against the smooth vinyl. I cried, but it wasn't the normal crying I'm used to, a response to thinking, an eventual giving up on not crying. It was abject and passive and barely connected to my brain at all; it was the crying I'm always warning my students against writing in their stories. "Tears filled my eyes." "Tears rolled down my cheeks." Tears pasted my face to the cushion.

The next morning Mom told me she'd heard the birthing women and crying babies, too. "I'm sorry," she said. "This is horrible." She blamed Suffolk—how stupid and backward it was to put all the women in the same part of the hospital, like some kind of red tent of suffering.

Suffering certainly happened there, but it wasn't a red tent or a place of shame. The maternity ward, like the one at the hospital where my support group met, was front and center: the one place in a hospital where people are supposed to be glad to go. That some people enter or leave a maternity ward terrified, alone, hurting, or in sorrow is not something we talk about. That the experience of maternity might cause someone to return decades later for surgery to repair the damage, and that a maternity ward might be a painful place for some of us, are other omissions of our culture.

But today Mom was feeling better. She could sit up and eat a little breakfast, rolled to her on a tray. Nurses came and went; they took her blood pressure and her temperature. She was in good shape to leave, the nurse said, if she felt as though we could handle things at home. *Oh definitely,* we both said. They began the process of discharging her.

Then another woman in scrubs came in, a large camera

fitted with a flash slung around her neck. She smiled at Mom. "Where's the baby?" she asked. "They always take them to the nursery right before I get there . . ."

Mom, who loves to be carded and didn't mind that time the policeman thought she was a child, smiled and waved. "I'm the baby!" she said.

"There is no baby," I explained.

It's strange to feel jealous of someone in the excruciating pain of labor, someone you can't see and don't know. I would not have traded places with a laboring woman in Suffolk, Virginia, but, like my friend the biologist, I thought it was unfair that I would not pass into the same community of human experience. Adrienne Rich wrote in her diary of jealousy—another silence we maintain as women, the reality of our own envy—directed at "the barren woman who has the luxury of her regrets but lives a life of privacy and freedom." She eventually repudiated the term "barren woman" and only a paragraph later in her diary entry acknowledges the love she has for her children, implicitly suggesting she'd never trade places with the childless.

On my drive back to Walkerton, on another blazing-hot day, I told Richard about my night in the hospital, how alienated and lonely I felt, and he reminded me that I couldn't know what got those women there. Maybe someone there had the same problems we had, he said. Maybe they tried IVF and now they had a child. "I doubt it," I said. I didn't want his reasonable or positive perspective.

I bought Kotex for my mom, and groceries. I stayed a few days, cooking and doing laundry and watching reruns of *Fashion Police* with her. We didn't talk about our time in Suffolk, the surgery or the maternity ward or whether she would ever be a grandmother. We didn't talk about what might be wrong with me or wrong with her.

"Mothers and daughters have always exchanged with each

other—beyond the verbally transmitted lore of female survival—a knowledge that is subliminal, subversive, preverbal,"
Rich writes in what she describes as the "core" of her memoir, the hardest and most crucial chapter. "[It is] the knowledge flowing between two alike bodies, one of which has spent
nine months inside the other." Rich describes women who have
powerful mental connections to their mothers in labor or who
suddenly remember the smell of their mother when they breast-
feed their own children. Menstruation, too, is an initiation into
the rites of womanhood. But what about the subverted body—
the one that doesn't bleed on schedule, doesn't endure labor
or suckle an infant? What about the aging female body? The
hospitalized female body? What about the body that isn't alike
in some way, the body that strays from the trajectory of womanhood through motherhood?

A fractious and eccentric mother-daughter pair once lived
next to my family in Walkerton—Miss Anne, the matriarch
of the family, and Miss Deirdre, her funny, profane daughter
("God*damn* it, Mama!" is the phrase I most associate with the
younger woman). After they died, we found a laundry hamper
in the pole barn behind their empty house stuffed with Miss
Deirdre's party dresses—frothy pastel ball gowns, strapless and
uncomfortably boned. Mom and I aired them on the clothesline
and kept them in a closet, for costumes and household decoration.

The day after we came home from Suffolk, I tried them all
on, sucking in and zipping up, flouncing around the scattered
cat dishes on their deck. Mom rested on the chaise longue
in a purple hat, a yellow nightgown, and Mardi Gras beads.
I wrapped my hair in a scarf like Little Edie in *Grey Gardens,*
draped myself in costume jewelry. We took turns holding the
tamest of Mom's eleven cats—Tadpole and Hush Puppy, just
kittens then—and snapping pictures.

I look back on the photos now and see my mother, an eccentric woman with two children, who has given paintings and

sculptures away all her life, who dreamed of being a doting grandmother like her beloved Donna, who feeds and spays and neuters all the stray cats in her town, who frightened me as a child by writing checks to "Shitty Bank" and claiming that communism didn't sound so bad by comparison with capitalism. Who has never been to Europe but sometimes talks about going with me. Who sleeps on seven down pillows and has a horror of gum chewing. Who keeps portfolios stuffed with every piece of paper my brother and I ever gave her. Whose mother kept a similar collection in her bedroom wardrobe. Whose mother died and left her alone—except that she had a daughter.

And there I am, hidden behind sunglasses and crinolines and kittens, someone who faints when she has blood drawn and was never any good at sports, who dreamed of having two kids like her mother but has been to Europe, who has published a book, has been a favorite and least-favorite teacher, a dutiful if sometimes less-than-useful daughter. In the background: a garden overgrown with zinnias and black-eyed Susans, pink crape myrtle blossoms strewn like confetti. It's so humid I can feel the thick, hot air fogging my sunglasses when I look at the photos, so familiar that I know, by slant of light, exactly the time of day.

It's eleven in the morning on August 9, seven days before my mother's sixty-second birthday, eight days before my tenth wedding anniversary. We look young in the photos, and healthy.

Visible Life

• • •

Among couples trying to conceive (or TTC, as it's known among people who have been trying for a while), there is something called the Two-Week Wait—the wait between ovulation and a positive or negative pregnancy test. Online message boards are filled with advice about what to do during the Two-Week Wait—go to the movies or out to dinner, take a yoga class, get a massage, anything to get your mind off the question of pregnancy. Richard and I were fond of walks to the river near our house, but we have never been good at taking our minds off anything. For a while, particularly when we were treating our infertility with oral medications and intrauterine insemination, it seemed as though every river walk involved a conversation about *what if:* What if this is the month? What if our child is born in January, February, March? The months flew by, forty-seven of them, and it was time to make decisions about our next step.

Instead of going to yoga or a movie, I visited an embryologist in her university laboratory during one of these Two-Week Waits. It had become clear to me, to Richard, and to our reproductive endocrinologist that IVF was the treatment most likely to overcome our infertility. But there were big questions: about the cost, about how we would feel if we tried and failed, about the ethical considerations of expending so many resources creating a life that has not happened naturally.

Even though IVF is still relatively uncommon, a treatment pursued by less than 5 percent of infertile couples, everyone seems to have an opinion about it—what it does to the woman's body, what one should do with leftover embryos, whether the treatment should be covered by insurance companies. Rational, loving friends and family told me all kinds of unhelpful things: that a child I conceived through IVF would be more likely to have autism; that IVF would give me cancer; that I would be better off with acupuncture, herbs, or drinking more whole milk.

So it shouldn't be surprising that politicians, who see a potent story written in petri dishes containing just a few cells, are involved in the debate. In 1972, arguing before the United States Supreme Court on behalf of pseudonymous appellant Jane Roe, attorney Sarah Weddington was asked whether a fetus could be given personhood status and what would happen to her argument then. "I would have a very difficult case," she allowed. Writing for the majority in the court's 1973 opinion, Justice Harry Blackmun noted that the court could find no such status but also allowed: "If this suggestion of personhood is established, [Roe's] case, of course, collapses, for the fetus' right to life would then be guaranteed."

This perceived loophole—fetal or even embryonic personhood—has been the driving force behind recent efforts to outlaw abortion and the motivator behind fetal homicide statutes, criminal prosecutions of drug-addicted pregnant women, and even the practice of issuing death certificates to stillborn babies. Before the 2012 Republican presidential convention, Personhood USA challenged Republican presidential candidates to sign a pledge to protect human life "at every stage of development." Five of seven candidates—Rick Santorum, Michele Bachmann, Newt Gingrich, Ron Paul, and Rick Perry—signed the pledge, and Gingrich, a converted Catholic, expressed concerns specifically about IVF: "If you have in vitro fertilization you are creating life; therefore we should look seriously at what should the rules be for clinics that are doing that, because they are creating life."

"I bet a lot of politicians have never stepped into an IVF clinic," said Dr. Silvia Ramos, a senior embryologist at the University of North Carolina School of Medicine, when I asked her about the personhood debate Gingrich was referencing. Born in Brazil, Dr. Ramos speaks with an accent that becomes more pronounced when she gets excited, and nearly everything about her work—from treating and interacting with patients to performing research on mouse ovaries—excites her. But about politicizing her lab, she was dismissive: "You need to have an understanding of science to know what goes on here. You need to have biological knowledge."

My biological knowledge about embryo development was rusty, mostly composed of half-remembered facts from school, but Dr. Ramos patiently and enthusiastically described the process of IVF, which begins when she receives the eggs retrieved from a woman's ovaries by the reproductive endocrinologist. In a sterile laboratory, she observes each egg, or oocyte, under a microscope and determines if it is mature enough for fertilization. If the patient has elected to undergo intracytoplasmic sperm injection, a procedure designed to overcome male infertility, Ramos will carefully remove the cloudy masses of nurse cells surrounding each mature oocyte and will inject the oocyte with a single sperm selected for optimum morphology and motility. This process can take an hour or more, and often she will listen to Brazilian bossa nova CDs as she works. "You have to be in peace every day to do your best at this," Ramos said. "Music helps."

After so many months of TTC, I found Ramos's step-by-step description soothing, even appealing, for its order and predictability, for the way it makes conception—that long-elusive goal—visible. If the oocyte is fertilized, Ramos will see the formation of two pronuclei, then the fusion of the diploid cell, or zygote. Over the next few days, as the zygote is incubated at thirty-seven degrees Celsius, she will track its development in the lab. Ideally, the zygote will form four even, smooth cells, then eight. If a number of healthy-looking embryos remain on day three, Ramos can wait for the best embryo to become a morula, which looks like a blackberry, or a blastula, which looks like a soccer ball, before transferring it to the woman's uterus (generally, embryologists and reproductive endocrinologists have the best chance of choosing the healthiest embryos when they wait until the blastula stage). "Look! How beautiful!" Ramos said, showing me images of embryos she had worked with. She had folders and folders full of these images, and they were, at every stage, strangely beautiful, as were her tools: the polished-steel-and-glass catheter used to collect the embryos, the tiny, needlelike cryoloop used to gather the leftover embryos for vitrification.

"What happens here in my laboratory is a lot like what happens in the woman's body," said Ramos. "No one sees it."

Except they do. The day of transfer to the uterus, Ramos gives each couple or individual a set of images of their embryo or embryos, plus a description of the embryos' condition and likelihood of implantation. I can imagine that these blobby, black-and-white images are precious to anyone who has experienced years of trying. Women on TTC message boards, women with screen names like Babybound or Tryn2BMommy, will send each other "sticky vibes" or "baby dust" in the hope the embryos will "take."

But in the clinic patients express only a cautious optimism. Sometimes they cry, Ramos said, but she has never seen her patients name or otherwise personify the embryos. There are too many things that can go wrong—the embryos, still months from viability, may not implant, or they may implant but stop developing. Extra embryos are frozen, and patients at her clinic have three options: they can store the embryos for future tries, they can donate them for research purposes, or they can destroy them. Destruction of a stored embryo is accomplished by thawing. "The embryos belong to the parents," said Ramos. "They have the right to decide."

And they are the ones who know, ultimately, the impact and import of IVF, a treatment that is so expensive, invasive, and fraught that it is rarely—if ever—begun lightly or heedlessly. Dr. Ramos often has to call her patients to give them disappointing, even devastating, news: embryos, especially those from the oocytes of older women, sometimes fragment or stop developing, and it is difficult to tell which ones will implant successfully. Despite this uncertainty, Ramos's discussion of IVF was punctuated by frequent, enthusiastic exclamations about the great love she has for her job. "It's so delicate," she said. "It takes the right combination of skill and personality to do it well. I create life. This is what is magic."

I looked up from the notebook where I'd been writing and sketching zygotes—*Did she say she creates life?*—but then Ramos went on to talk about the life of the family: mothers and fathers and children, or mothers and mothers, or fathers and fathers, birthdays and holidays, traditions passed on, one generation to another. That is the life she helps create, the life she or another embryologist offers me and Richard.

Near the end of my visit, our conversation turned from the theoretical consideration of morulas and blastulas to the specific realities of my own condition and treatment. Very politely, Dr. Ramos asked my age, and I told her. "Now is your time," she said.

She was probably right, I thought. Our Two-Week Wait was over, and—as I had come to expect—Richard and I were still TTC. Visiting Dr. Ramos did not answer my questions about money or the use of resources or the exposure to heartbreak. But in my waiting moments, in the space of *what if?* I could picture myself receiving a phone call from her. *Beautiful embryos,* I pictured her saying, a bossa nova melody playing in the background. I pictured the embryos themselves: round blastulas with evenly divided cells.

Though even then, we would still be waiting.

The word *obstetrician,* my reproductive endocrinologist wrote in an email, has as its Latin morphemes *ob,* which means "across," and *stare,* which means "to stand." An obstetrician is someone who stands across from his patient, waiting to bring forth her child. (And then there is that word *patient,* and all that it implies.)

Dr. Young waits, too, but in a different way. He diagnoses and treats long periods of waiting, and he waits for women like me—waffling, indecisive, fearful—to decide what to do. When his patients become and stay pregnant, they eventually "graduate" to an obstetrician, who will be the one to deliver their babies. Dr. Young waits for the correct combination of treatments to take effect—he waits, like us, for the pregnancy.

I was diagnosed by Dr. Young with a luteal phase defect, meaning that my endometrium, my uterine lining, does not wait long enough before shedding each month. For a time this was treated through progesterone supplements, which I took after ovulation. My cycle became a regular twenty-eight days, and my endometrium waited properly—two full weeks—for the blastula to implant.

Except that it didn't. I didn't get pregnant—at least, I never confirmed a pregnancy through a positive e.p.t. or First Response testing kit. In fact, I had taken very few pregnancy tests in my years of reproductive maturity—once when Richard and I were living in Brooklyn, and three times in the forty-seven months we'd been trying. Instead I took my temperature every morning, and usually, near the end of my cycle, I would see a pattern of falling temperatures—98.5, 98.3, 98.2—that told me the Two-Week Wait was nearly over.

In this way I was unusual. On message boards and in the support group I attended, TTC women talked about testing daily, even twice a day, during their Two-Week Wait. Sometimes they were waiting for a positive result—usually, the soonest that home pregnancy tests can detect hCG in a woman's urine is ten days past ovulation—but other times they were confirming and reconfirming a positive result. I'd heard of women taking two or three tests to prove—to celebrate?—what one test showed: the dark line, the plus sign, the word *Pregnant.*

I could well understand that this was comforting to them in the same way that Dr. Ramos's evenly dividing embryo cells were to me. Because the embryo and the changes to the body are longed for, expected, and (at this point) invisible, a TTC woman desires anything that makes the pregnancy seem real. Of course, she might not share this information publicly, but among her TTC cohorts, other women who are waiting to hear the results of her treatment, she will probably share. Online, such news might be delivered through an exultation—"Yippee!!! BFP!" (big, fat positive)—or an image: a photograph of the home pregnancy test, or a smiley-faced icon of a pregnant woman holding her rounded belly.

Infertility and assisted reproduction can be difficult to talk about with fertile people—they may not understand, may not want to talk about it, or may be too busy raising their own families to offer much support. A message board or blog is a safe place to talk about injectable medications, IVF cycles, or the question that plagues every Two-Week Waiter, no matter how many movies she sees: *Am I pregnant—or not?* Though mediated through a computer, the support offered by women on these boards is conversational—filled with sentence fragments, terms of endearment, urgent questions, and exuberant punctuation. Their messages are decorated with animated GIFs that are like body language or gestures in a face-to-face conversation:

cartwheeling or cheerleading smiley faces, illuminated BFPs, shimmering baby dust.

On the website Lilypie.com, a TTC woman can create a custom ticker—a colorful graphic image that counts up or down—to appear below her posts to infertility and assisted-reproduction message boards. As I visited these boards, I often saw, below a list of relevant details—ages, medical conditions, number of months or years TTC, the dates and results of various IUI or IVF cycles—these small, rectangular banners, frequently more up-to-date than the posts themselves.

Tickers can provide a digital reminder of all kinds of things—vacations, anniversaries, birthdays, and graduations are all popular events to anticipate via ticker—but they have a particular significance and prevalence in the infertility community, where conception and pregnancy are marked by a series of emotionally fraught, unseen events that might be shared only in anonymous places such as Internet message boards. Like medieval manuscripts, the tickers are illuminated with images that represent the text, pastel pictures you might see on any baby shower invitation: infant clothes, a pram, smiling cartoon storks. On Lilypie, you can choose to mark a menstrual cycle from fifteen to eighty days long, using a variety of backgrounds: butterflies, the city at night, a cabbage patch, or stars. (Fertile days in a cycle might be marked with hearts or a sprinkling of baby dust.) The "slider" is the image that will mark where you are in the cycle, and it's customizable, too; choices include a gleeful rabbit, a woman jumping through a hoop, or a variety of cartoon pairings: bees, ladybugs, a man and a woman holding hands, two women holding hands, or two men holding hands (presumably marking a surrogate's cycle).

There are also "angel baby" memorial tickers for children lost to miscarriage or stillbirth. Backgrounds include clouds, rainbows, and serene meadows, and sliders include doves, teddy bears, bunnies, and babies of various ethnicities and postures:

some are sleeping peacefully, while others are sitting upright and are haloed, heaven bound. Some have wings, some slide down rainbows; they come in singles or groups of two, three, or four. They all look the way we expect babies, not embryos, to look; they are pleasantly chubby, adorably forelocked, dressed in shades of blue or pink. The suggested message for an angel-baby ticker is "It's been x months & y days since we said good-bye." The grieving mother might have lost her baby at birth or sometime long before—with IVF, losses are common days or weeks after the transfer of embryos. Though books may tell her that her baby at three to four weeks is the size of a poppy seed, that is not what she pictures. She imagines a "real" baby: smiling, gendered, and cuddly. But the angel baby—a cartoon, an image, an idea—might be all she gets.

Before we had the technology we have now—before home pregnancy tests, before IVF, before microscopic images of blastulas—a pregnancy was suspected with a missed period, but imminent life was confirmed not through a visual sign but through the quickening, the first fetal movements felt by the mother, which typically happens at four or five months' gestation. Aristotle considered quickening the signal that a human soul had entered the fetus. Until about a hundred years ago, when doctors and scientists began collecting and displaying fetal specimens, most people could not picture an embryo or a fetus—and didn't try. In some cultures, fetuses born very prematurely were so foreign and unfamiliar that they were interpreted as something other than human—as kangaroos, monkeys, fish bellies, or spirits.

It is now possible, in the most advanced and high-tech reproductive endocrinology clinics, to record every moment of cell division in an IVF cycle through time-lapse imaging. Embryologists believe that by studying these images—how and when each embryo divides—they will be able to select the best-quality embryos for transfer, improving the patient's likelihood of pregnancy. Such images will surely become the subject of political and bioethical debates—the time-stamped creation of life is a powerful tool for those concerned with personhood at the cellular level. Dr. Ramos, for her part, is excited by the extra assurance this technology offers her patients and hopes to obtain it for her laboratory in the next few years. By then, we agreed, my decision will be made. I will have tried IVF. Or I will have moved on.

Just Adopt

. . .

Nate and Parul Goetz had recently come home from their baby shower, a surprise event at Nate's office, when Parul got the call from the adoption agency. An economist at a social-services non-profit in the Raleigh area, Nate described the shower as so "incredibly awkward and weird"—there was no baby or due date yet—that he'd gone out with a friend for drinks while Parul sorted through their gifts and took the unexpected call.

It was an unusual situation, she was told. The child, a boy, had been born five weeks prematurely just days ago. Kate, his birth mother, was on her way to Utah—home of the adoption agency and laws giving birth mothers only twenty-four hours to change their minds—when she went into labor and delivered at a rural Indiana hospital. Soon after, she was transferred to a better-equipped hospital in Kentucky. Kate had seen Parul and Nate's profile and had chosen them to be her son's parents—they could say yes or no, but if they wanted to adopt him, they needed to be there the next day, the agency representative told Parul, and prepared to stay in Kentucky for the three weeks it would take to complete the process.

Parul started packing immediately, stuffing armloads of unwashed baby clothes, the bounty of their well-timed shower, into suitcases. She and Nate left at three the next morning and were in Kentucky by the following afternoon.

It was July 2010. In April and May, they'd spent weeks creating the family profile they hoped would appeal to someone like Kate: writing the story of their lives, describing their home and community in North Carolina, taking photographs of Parul gardening and Nate golfing. Parul tried to put herself in the birth mother's shoes, imagining what she might want to know about the life her child would lead with them.

But it wasn't the carefully constructed life story that mattered to Kate, a twenty-three-year-old woman who first gave birth at fourteen and, with limited resources and education, had adopted her other children out to members of her extended family. North Carolina law permits birth mothers—wherever they're from—access to home studies completed there, and Kate had requested and read Nate and Parul's. She was struck by a strange symmetry in their lives—she'd had six children before this baby, and Parul had had six miscarriages. This baby—her seventh—was also Parul's seventh attempt at a family. It seemed fated.

It's compelling to think that if you don't have luck conceiving a child, perhaps fate has something else in store for you. After Richard and I stopped IUI treatment, I thought that maybe I was *meant to adopt*—that's the way I thought of it, as the revelation of some long-obscured plan.

In *Blue Nights,* Joan Didion describes the adoption of her daughter with an emphasis on its mythic elements. Like the Goetzes, Didion and her husband, John Gregory Dunne, had little time to decide whether they wanted to claim the child waiting in the hospital, and they also said yes right away. They named her Quintana Roo, after a territory they'd seen on a map in Mexico a few months earlier, when the idea of a daughter, adopted or otherwise, was "dreamy speculation." They'd never been to the rural territory—"The place on the map called Quintana Roo was still terra incognita," Didion writes. But they didn't hesitate when the hospital asked what her name would be. They knew right away, just as they knew that the child described to them over the phone as a "beautiful baby girl at St. John's" was the very child they wanted.

I never pictured a newborn or the birth mother, but I thought about what it might be like to have a four-year-old, a six-year-old, a ten-year-old. I drew on my experiences as a teacher, the bonds I had with children who weren't genetically related to me. I thought especially of my first-grade student Daniel Hall, his face so full of sunshine I could send him anywhere in our dilapidated school building, and he'd come back with precious supplies: photocopies or pencils from the office manager, snacks from the cafeteria workers, chalk or markers from a neighboring teacher. My heart sank on the few days he wasn't there to greet me in the breakfast line; I'd agreed to teach first grade, a shift from my role as a writing teacher to the whole school, only if Daniel would be in my class. I knew if he was there, I could tolerate anything: our laborious and impossible bathroom process (we had to stand single file in the hallway, completely silent, while the children took turns one by one), the increased paperwork pressure and additional scrutiny from a principal we called Darth Vader.

How great it would be to skip the hard, boring infant years and move right into the things I knew about: reading Ezra Jack Keats and decorating our house with messy art projects, riding bicycles and going to museums. Worries about advanced maternal age would disappear—I'd be young as the mother of a six-year-old! And perhaps I'd be a better mother to a child not genetically related to me, I thought, more accepting and careful. I wouldn't see my own faults written in his behavior.

But Daniel had two loving parents, and when I imagined adopting someone like him, I was conjuring a fantasy. The adopted and foster children I'd taught were often troubled beyond my help or their parents'—they refused to come to school, acted out, were suspended. A few years after teaching Daniel's class, I had an AP English student who struggled—despite her intelligence and her loving, well-resourced home, she found it so emotionally difficult to come to school that she accrued too many absences to graduate. At the beginning of the year, before her truancy began, she frequently spoke or wrote about her adoption and the lingering scars she carried from being neglected and unwanted. I was shocked when I learned that she was only eight months old when she was adopted.

Adoption, whenever it takes place, is traumatic for someone involved: the birth mother or father, the bewildered new parents, the child. Sometimes all of them. Yet it is also a powerful, attractive narrative, especially in the face of infertility. Look up any list of things not to say to infertile couples, and you'll find the suggestion "You should just adopt"—we've heard it, and read it, and probably even thought it ourselves. There are so many children in the world who need homes, the story goes, millions of them. To focus on your loss, your inability to become pregnant or have a genetically related child, is selfish.

I liked imagining myself as an adoptive mother. I signed up for a foster-adopt class, scanned adoption blogs, and researched the international programs with the shortest wait times and the lowest in-country fees. Richard, initially skeptical, found it hard to argue with my reasoning: if adoption depends on completing paperwork and telling stories about your life, wouldn't we, two writers, have a better-than-average chance at success? I imagined us convincing a social worker that our long marriage and my work as a public school teacher would make us ideal adoptive parents. I thought about giving up the expensive, unpleasant treatments for good and turning to a series of steps over which we'd at least have some control. I saw us passing a test my body had failed.

For a while I thought we'd adopt from Ethiopia, but then ethical concerns about that country's surging program emerged, and officials there halted new adoptions. Perhaps Haiti would be better—we met with an agency that processed Haitian adoptions, and I spoke to a woman who'd adopted a Haitian daughter. But the agency couldn't assure us that the same thing that happened in Ethiopia would not happen in Haiti, another country with rumors of coercive, unethical practices and a sudden spike in adoptions from the United States.

In my support group, we talked occasionally about adoption, sharing news about programs we considered favorable—wait times less than two years, comparatively low fees, a chance of adopting an infant. I told the group I'd read that you could get a newborn from Morocco in about a year. A couple of women leaned forward: *And?*

You have to get an in-country medical exam, I explained. *And convert to Islam, if you're not Muslim.*

I'd brought up Moroccan adoptions as a way of joking about our desperation, and people laughed. But the truth was, I'd thought about it—imagined myself getting religion at thirty-five and also deceiving a foreign government with a fake conversion. Either way I'd be a mother, the experience of religiosity or deception, or deception that turned religious, integrated into the story of my family.

Parul and Nate Goetz didn't know about RESOLVE when they were struggling with infertility, though "it would have been useful," Nate said. I actually met them through RESOLVE—they visited my support group to talk about the foundation they started in 2011, which seeks to educate infertile couples about domestic adoption and provide financial assistance to couples adopting after unsuccessful infertility treatment. At the time they were meeting with couples and small groups in their home, for free, to provide Domestic Adoption 101, an introductory course, and Domestic Adoption 102, a more intensive overview.

Before they adopted, Nate and Parul spent years under a reproductive endocrinologist's care: first with Clomid cycles, then with IUI. Together and individually they saw a psychologist at Duke Fertility, and they attended an eight-week-long support group with other couples in treatment there. By then, after six miscarriages in five years, they'd stopped treatment and were the only couple in the group who did not conceive.

Parul said that after their last loss, twins, she'd finally come to accept that fertility treatments would not work and that what she'd always imagined as a happy experience—starting a family—was becoming unsustainably stressful. Still, it was hard for her to give up on trying. She had a doctorate of pharmacy and a lot of responsibility at her job as a pharmacology scientist. "At this point in my life," she said, "I'd never had a failure."

They'd been mostly silent with family and friends about their repeat miscarriages and their fear they might never have a child. When Parul's younger sister, one of the only people she'd told about their fertility problems, gave birth in Los Angeles, Parul found out through a call from her father. She'd had no idea that her sister was pregnant.

Parul flew to be with her sister and meet her niece the next day. Though her sister had thought she was protecting Parul's feelings, Parul was hurt by the decision she made to keep the birth secret. "All the emotions of wanting to be a mom and not being a mom came out," she told me, recounting how hard she felt she was, in retrospect, on her sister. She bossed her about breast-feeding and nutrition, all the things she'd read about and planned for her child. I thought of my own childless time in a maternity ward with my mother: how lonely I felt, how separate from other women, but also how ready to make a decision, to stop living in the liminal space of child*less.* Parul came home to North Carolina a week later and talked to Nate about what they truly wanted: a child, they decided, whether or not it was genetically related to them.

We were sitting together in their living room, a comfortable but minimally decorated space where Nate and Parul met with other couples to give their Domestic Adoption 101 and 102 seminars. Aldo, their dog, snored in a corner; Noah, the son they adopted at one week old, was at preschool.

"When we were trying, we tried to imagine what the child would look like," Parul said. "You invest in that concept."

"You become trapped in it," Nate added.

Isolated from most everyone outside the clinic, Parul and Nate didn't know anyone who'd gone through something like their experience, and by the time they decided to pursue adoption, they didn't know anyone from that world either. They hired a consultant who talked them through the steps of adoption during a series of phone conversations. They completed a home study and selected an agency, then began compiling the adoptive-family profile the agency would use to match them with a birth mother. But the night they matched and had to decide to travel to Kentucky—it was only six weeks after completing the paperwork—their consultant, who'd charged them $2,500, was on vacation and unavailable.

Parul and Nate don't regret any decisions that led them to their son, but they note the emotional distance they felt from the consultant, who told them *I'm not a therapist,* as if deflecting any claim on her empathy.

"The information was good, but it was also just business," Parul said.

"[The adoption business] has very little empathy, and that's a problem," Nate added. "You're talking about three different people: the birth mother, the child, the adoptive parents. It requires a great deal of empathy."

This perceived lack of empathy was one inspiration for their foundation—they thought they could do better than the impersonal, businesslike, and piecemeal approach they'd found with their consultant. Another inspiration was a desire to pay homage to their son's birth mother. "We were so moved by her selfless act of love," Parul said. "We asked ourselves, 'How can we give thanks?'"

They send photos and letters describing their son's life to the adoption agency; she can choose to collect them or get in touch. But mostly, they don't hear from her.

Most primate babies are semiprecocial—not as helpless at birth as a baby rabbit or rat is, but requiring a lot of costly caretaking— and also attractive not only to their mothers but to other members of their species. This can work out well for mothers, who may need to hand off their infants while foraging, and sometimes less well for babies, who are occasionally kidnapped by ill-prepared but highly interested adolescents. Primate mothers have even been documented as oblivious or insensitive to an accidental switch. And zookeepers will often place primate infants with adoptive mothers, either to broaden the gene pool of a breeding group or when a birth mother rejects her infant.

Human parents usually require help, from grandparents, family and friends, day cares and schools. It's hard to imagine human families without the recourse of adoption—there is no guarantee we'll live long enough to see our offspring safely to adulthood or that some other misfortune won't separate birth parents and their children. In the United States alone, some 120,000 adoptions are completed each year, about double the number of births by IVF. Of parents seeking to adopt, three-quarters are infertile or subfertile.

Still, adoption can be as frightening an unknown—Didion's "terra incognita"—as the process of assisted reproduction. We've all heard the nightmare stories of adoptions that go wrong for the birth mother, the child, the parents-to-be. Nate and Parul told me one: Two clients pursued an adoption with an unvetted domestic adoption agency. The birth mother, who chose the adoptive parents and completed the relinquishment period, neglected to tell them that the child's father was in prison. The agency neglected to determine his whereabouts. Maybe the birth mother thought that because he was in prison he had no rights, but he was released, and he did. He claimed the child, against the wishes of the birth mother and to the despair of the adoptive parents she had chosen.

Stories like this one have long made domestic adoption a fearful choice for the infertile, who perceive the risk of emotional trauma and financial loss as too similar to what they have already endured in the fertility clinic. Often, we have become so used to failure that we accept it as our due, so self-focused that we define it only in relation to our own experience. Of course something will go wrong—the birth mother will change her mind, will want the child back after we have held him, fed him, fallen in love with him.

This is one reason that for the past couple of decades so many American adoptive parents have been drawn to international adoption. By the 1990s, better access to contraception, a lower teen birthrate, and decreased social stigma surrounding unmarried parenting meant that fewer American-born infants were available. International adoption looked simpler and less expensive, with far more infants available; by the year 2000, U.S. adoptions from other countries had doubled, to about twenty thousand a year. (Because of ethical concerns over programs such as the ones Richard and I researched, that number has since been cut by more than half.) The children were presented as orphans in need of a home; their surviving family members, if they had any, were presumably too poor and far away to take them back. These family members would be grateful to have their children raised in a prosperous country like

America, and in a few years the child could return for a tour of her birth country.

My friends Mark and Rachel Alexander saw adoption as the best way to add to their family when they began the process of adopting Dejen, their son, who was born in Ethiopia. Rachel had a miscarriage at age thirty-nine and was more attracted to adoption than to assisted reproduction. She had a close colleague who had adopted from Ethiopia and who recommended *There Is No Me without You,* a book by Melissa Fay Greene that detailed the plight of thousands of children in Ethiopia orphaned by the HIV/AIDS epidemic. Mark and Rachel, who live in the progressive mountain community of Asheville, North Carolina, looked forward not only to another child in the family but also to becoming a multicultural family. Mark is a photographer interested in endangered landscapes, Rachel a family physician who specializes in transgender health and HIV care.

"When you get into it you think it's a kind of pure thing, to help some little boy or girl whose parents are dead or unable to take care of them, and at the same time to have the larger family you want. Everybody wins," Mark told me. "But of course it's more complicated than that."

At first they envisioned adopting a toddler, but the more Mark thought about the challenges of toddlerhood, and the age difference such a young child would share with Violet, their seven-year-old daughter, the more he was attracted to their agency's "waiting children"—kids slightly older or with special needs, who were considered harder to place. Scrolling through photos on the agency's website, Mark noticed a photo of a four-year-old boy with round cheeks and soft, brown curls, holding one hand over his chest. "He looks like a sweetie," Mark told his wife.

And he was. Just months later, after completing multiple rounds of paperwork, Mark and Rachel flew to Addis Ababa and went directly to the orphanage to meet Dejen. Children about to be adopted are prepared for the arrival of their new families with photos and reminders about the day they'll arrive. Dejen, who'd been playing with a group of children, jumped up and ran across the courtyard, leaping into their arms. "It was pretty wonderful," Mark said.

They spent the next couple of days with Dejen, then took him to the embassy to complete his adoption paperwork. On the fourth day, they left him at the orphanage and took a four-hour jeep trip into Awasa and another two-hour drive to Arbegona, the remote town closest to Dejen's birth family. They passed beautiful, rugged scenery that also gave them a glimpse of the poverty they'd read about: intricately woven reed huts, a field plowed by a single ox dragging a sharpened eucalyptus limb. At a community center in Arbegona, they were introduced by their translator to the social worker who helped arrange the adoption and to Dejen's aunt and uncle, who cared for him before he went to live in the orphanage and had made a two-hour journey on foot to meet them. Such introductions are common—they create a sense of openness about the adoption process but also provide adoptive parents a chance to collect resources and information about their child's birth family. Mark took hundreds of photographs. Through the translator, he and Rachel asked about Dejen's birth mother. What was she like? Tall, they were told, with a great sense of humor. Everyone in town loved her. How did she die? They couldn't be sure; she was sick for a long time, and the nearest hospital was a prohibitive six-hour drive from their home. When Mark and Rachel returned to the hotel with other adoptive families, they were struck by the similarities of stories people had been told—so many birth mothers who were tall and lovable and funny. But, they reminded themselves, many people are remembered in general, glowing terms after they're gone.

Back home in Asheville, they settled into life as a family of four. Mark and Rachel put together a book of photographs of

Ethiopia and of Dejen's family, and when he got a little older, they would sit and talk to him about the way he became part of their life. *Your parents loved you very much,* they would tell him, *but they died.* And Dejen would say, *No, my parents didn't die. Well, yes, I'm sorry, they did,* they'd say. *No,* he always said. *My parents aren't dead.*

Eventually he told them that he believed the man and woman who'd presented themselves as his aunt and uncle were in fact his parents. Stories like this one were becoming common in Ethiopian adoptions—the presence of translators and corruption, the absence of documentation such as birth and death certificates, and overwhelming interest from wealthy countries made it hard to tell whether birth families were fully informed about the way Western-style adoptions work and whether the children were truly orphaned.

In 2014, Mark and Rachel hired an Ethiopian investigator, who traveled to Arbegona to look into Dejen's birth story but didn't discover anything definitive. They felt it was their responsibility to Dejen, but it's not like they would have sent him home—he's their son. A ten-year-old boy who loves soccer and books and remote control cars and is sometimes rigid and anxious. I remember visiting their house once for brunch and seeing a list of numbered rules, the sort you might see in a classroom, posted in the dining room. I learned later that the family had made the rules together as a way of making mealtimes more peaceful. "Dejen thrives at school," Mark explained, noting how in this way—with an insistence on schedules and clear expectations—he is temperamentally like Rachel but also a good match for Mark, who sees his own, more casual approach to life, his resistance to schedules and timelines, as a challenge he needs to work on for his whole family. "Dejen is the perfect boy for me to have to deal with my stuff as a person, as a human being," Mark said. "All my weaknesses."

Like all families, theirs is a work in progress. They go to

therapy, are part of an adoptive-family community, and in 2015 planned a summer trip to an Ethiopian culture camp in Virginia. For Dejen, thinking about his adoption and the loss of his original family, country, and culture, plus the simple fact that being born in Ethiopia makes him different from most of his peers, can be extremely stressful. Mark and Rachel try to honor Ethiopia's noble history and culture, but Mark also notes that their son is black, while Violet, Mark, and Rachel are white, and that makes for another kind of navigation.

"I was thinking, for instance, how if I was black I couldn't do what I do, which frequently is walk around neighborhoods pointing cameras at houses," Mark told me in an email. "And of course I worry for Dejen and for how difficult it will be, and already is, for him to navigate being black, and on top of that being in a white family.

"I remember feeling so in love with Dejen right away, and feeling so lucky to have him, but also feeling like the whole thing was a tragedy, even before we suspected that his aunt and uncle were actually his parents," he continued. "Maybe life is really just like that. Actually I'm pretty sure it is—and we don't really do what it takes to fix it."

I can picture Mark sitting in his garage studio while he writes this email, long panoramic photographs of blasted mountaintop-removal sites and West Virginia prison yards taped to the walls. In addition to landscapes and portraits, Mark makes aerial photography—he sends a tethered digital camera up a few hundred feet using a helium balloon and a remote control and snaps thousands of photos. Later he assembles them on his computer, fitting the images together into a single, completed puzzle. He is drawn, he says, to the paradox of the form, which he describes as "all-seeing, but [which] is also, by definition, impossible to take in." Too much information to process. For me the compressed, dizzying images are a little like Mark and Rachel's trip to Ethiopia and Dejen's trip back to America with them: pieced together with visible seams, like a quilt or a flag. Ragged at the edges.

We don't really do what it takes to fix it. What if all the money spent on international adoption went toward development in those countries—would the "aunts and uncles" of Ethiopia or Haiti be able to keep their children? What if the money spent on domestic adoption went to education and food and housing for birth mothers—would Kate, the young woman whose generosity inspired the Goetzes' foundation, have kept her baby? What if all the money spent on IVF went toward health care for the poor? Could I fund instead someone else's more direly needed reproductive care?

Adoption and IVF are often treated as radically opposed choices, each with their own separate virtues. The adoptive parents were not selfish; they used their resources to do some good. They saved a child and enlarged their own community. They saw beyond genetics, skin color, background. The IVF parents were maybe selfish but definitely lucky; they didn't have to get involved with anyone else's pain. In their child they see a mother's blue eyes, a grandfather's stubborn streak or gift for mathematics.

But look at the obstacles to both kinds of birth stories, and you'll see that there is a kinship between them. We might cheer the adoptive family or pity the fertility patient, but they are offered little in the way of the support that matters: a $13,400 federal tax credit, retroactive and nonrefundable, favors adoptive families of means and hardly covers the associated expenses. Most insurance plans cover few of the costs of fertility treatment.

And look closer: for people who reason that adoption is good because it means a woman did not abort her fetus, IVF can be seen negatively or positively. On the negative side, the IVF patient, like the abortion patient, is interfering with nature, with God's creation. She is exerting too much control when we expect her to take what comes, grasping through science instead of accepting with dignity and faith. But more positively, perhaps the extra embryos created in a cycle can be adopted, treated as "snowflake babies" whose home is selected by the original gamete bearers, rather than as collections of cells that might be donated to a fertility clinic or thawed when the patients no longer need them. By participating in the "adoption," the IVF patient and recipient parents-to-be wittingly or unwittingly bolster the argument that embryos are children.

And closer still: the adoptive family does not give up on genetic links after all. New research shows that we are natured by our nurture. The professor whose class in evolutionary biology I audited explained that we usually conceptualize genes as architects drawing blueprints. Instead, she suggested, think of genes as trucks pulling up to a loading dock, full of materials and waiting for instructions from lived experience. So a fruit fly's genetically coded number of bristles can be altered by water temperature at the pupal stage. And so, when a parent adopts, she is not merely accepting what someone else's genetic lottery hands her. She is part of that lottery too.

"It is unfortunate to hear the label 'biological mother' applied to a woman who has given birth to a child and given it up for adoption . . . ," writes Sarah Hrdy in *Mother Nature,* her book on maternal instinct. "Such a woman is more nearly the *genetic* or *gestational* mother. By contrast to a genetic donor, the *biological* mother nourishes, nurtures, and provides the environment in which the infant develops both physically and psychologically."

Even the brilliant Hrdy wades into tricky waters with her correction of *biological*—what about that phrase "given it up for adoption"? A birth mother I know, a talented young poet who had a daughter at twenty and still regularly communicates with both the child and her adoptive mothers, takes issue with *give up,* which implies a lack of care, choice, or agency. I asked her if *placed* sounded better, and she thought for a while before answering that there weren't any words that worked.

Like Frost ("Good fences make good neighbors") and Shakespeare ("Neither a borrower nor a lender be"), Joan Didion is sometimes misapprehended outside of context. "We tell ourselves stories in order to live," a quote from "The White Album," sounds to some like an argument for the importance and usefulness of storytelling; it is even the reassuring title of my Everyman's Library edition of her collected essays. But Didion isn't a reassuring writer, and "The White Album" isn't about the uplifting or salvational nature of stories—it's about the collapse of narrative, its utter uselessness in the face of chaos.

Following progressive adoptive parenting advice, Didion and Dunne created and retold a "choice narrative" for Quintana Roo, with Dunne describing the way he selected the beautiful baby girl with a ribbon tied in her dark hair ("Not *that* baby . . . *that* baby. The baby with the ribbon") and Didion describing the call from the doctor who delivered her, which came while she was in the shower. "Do *that* baby," Quintana would beg them. Or, "Tell the part about the shower."

Later, Didion realized that the narrative that she thought her child accepted and found solacing was also a source of anxiety: *"What if you hadn't answered the phone when Dr. Watson called,* she would suddenly say. *What if you hadn't been home, what if you couldn't meet him at the hospital, what if there'd been an accident on the freeway, what would happen to me then?"*

The story she told did not hold together; it was not sufficient to allay Quintana's fear of abandonment and instability, which began with her birth story. Didion wrote that after Quintana's official adoption, at seven months, she thought that fear had left them; only later did she realize that it would reside in her daughter forever. There is no such thing as an uncomplicated adoption, no matter how fortuitous it seems. No one *just* adopts, because no child is ever just adopted.

It is impossible for stories to protect us or to travel unchanged through time, but still we lean on them. Courting a sense of adoptive-parent fatedness was a way of claiming an identity that allowed me to feel lucky and special, possessed of a unique story instead of driven to last resort. I held on to it as a possibility for a long time, checking websites, reading blogs of happy families, scrolling through descriptions of kids with a love of animals or sports or nature, kids with glasses and toothy grins and cartoon-character T-shirts. A representative from the adoption agency I chose warned me that her agency preferred to work with people who were done with fertility treatment—it was too difficult, in their experience, to balance both pursuits at once. I told her we *were* done, for now, but the truth was, we weren't. As complicated and risky as IVF felt to me, I worried more about getting adoption wrong—choosing the wrong country or state, the wrong agency. So I never got far in the process, never completed a home study or enrolled in a foster-care class, never formally contracted with an adoption agency or paid any fees. I still get letters in the mail from my county's foster-care program. I recycle them guiltily but don't ask to be taken off the list.

Nate and Parul are careful to avoid the narrative of fate when talking to their clients, even though the perception of fate—six babies, six miscarriages—played a role in their adoption of the boy they named Noah.

"We tell people adoption isn't *the* way to build a family," Nate said. "It's *a* way."

They have clients who go on to adopt successfully and clients who return to IVF, donor-egg, or donor-embryo cycles and are successful that way. Some of their clients, even the ones who have not adopted, come back as volunteers or donors to their foundation. They attend potlucks and Halloween parties. The Goetzes, once isolated from other couples and families, now have a wide circle of friends who know what it means to wait for the life they wanted.

All families start as stories, however true or untrue they become. A person has something in mind—a refrigerator covered in bright tempera paintings, a whole afternoon watching frogs in a pond. Board books chewed at their edges. Mispronounced words. Accidental wisdom. Milky breath. The tooth fairy. Ballet recitals. Time standing still and time moving too quickly. A community of people who feel the same. Feeling the same as the community.

The life an infertile person seeks comes to her not by accident and not by fate but by hard-fought choices. How to put together the portfolio of photographs. How to answer at the home study. What clinic or doctor or procedure. Donor egg or donor sperm or donor embryo. Open or closed adoption. What country, what boxes to check or uncheck. What questions to ask, and ask again. When to start and when to stop.

What to say when her child says, *Tell me my story.*

Solstice

• • •

Our last two years as a childless couple, Richard and I spent our winter holidays far from home and family.

In 2011, we drove to Florida to stay in the gulfside condo of a family friend. On the day we arrived, we headed to the beach to watch the pink and orange sunset. The curving expanse of cool white sand, sparsely populated just an hour before, was suddenly filled with people, some of them carrying beach chairs and blankets, some of them with cameras. There were Mennonites in long skirts and bonnets, hippies with bongo drums, retirees with deep winter tans. "It's the solstice," I told Richard. We found a space to ourselves and watched the long show of brilliant, then fading, light. I was glad to think that for the next six months, each day would be a little longer. Already, because of the difference in latitude, the days were longer here than they were at home.

But the next evening, and every night for the rest of our vacation, the same people arrived at around the same time, and so did we. During the day we did things we didn't do at home—slept late, watched John Grisham movies, wandered the beach looking for shells. And every night, we watched the sun disappear. In the elevator of the condo building, a photocopied notice described what some of the sunset watchers must have been looking for: the green flash, an optical phenomenon in which a bright-green spot or ray appears momentarily at sunrise or sunset. The notice mentioned the novel *The Green Ray* by Jules Verne, which popularized the superstition that anyone who sees the green flash will experience good luck and insight.

The following year I didn't want sunsets and beach weather but darkness, trolls, glaciers—so we booked a trip to Iceland.

It should have been a hopeful time. In late summer and into the fall, I'd exchanged emails with Dr. Young about possible start dates for our first IVF cycle. August was too soon, September and October taken up with travel for work. "I'm the Hamlet of assisted reproduction," I told him. "Endlessly debating, endlessly putting off the inevitable." (I was grateful when he didn't remind me about the ending of *Hamlet.*)

I didn't mean only the inevitability of IVF, but also its finality. There was no other procedure we could afford after paying for our medication and treatment, not donor egg or donor embryo. Our investigation of adoption, too, had been complicated and uncertain.

We thought that the Iceland trip would take our minds off things. We planned to arrive two days before the solstice and hoped amid that darkness we'd see the aurora borealis, that display of shimmering, multicolored photons that often can be seen on clear nights. Cultures all over the world have built mythology around auroras—the Chinese said they were dragons; the Cree believed that they were ancestral spirits. In Iceland, where a majority of people still profess faith in elves, the lights are thought to ease the pains of childbirth.

I imagined that the northern lights would communicate something to me, five years into my unhappy childlessness. Maybe something about the universe's capacity for beauty and surprise, or a peace with things as they are. Maybe insight. I imagined myself standing atop a glacier on the shortest day of the year, looking up.

I'd spent the summer and fall reporting a story I couldn't get out of my head, about people who'd lived almost their whole lives knowing they couldn't reproduce. They weren't infertile but had been surgically sterilized by my home state as part of our now-defunct, and long-ago discredited, eugenics program. North Carolina was one of thirty-three states to pass eugenics legislation, using forced and coercive sterilization to decide who should and should not become parents. Our sterilization program began in 1933 and continued into the 1970s. As in other states, the program targeted minorities and the poor, often pressuring the guardians of children suspected of promiscuity or mental deficits to consent to sterilization. *If you don't consent, you'll have your welfare benefits taken away,* parents and grandparents were threatened.

Willis Lynch, a veteran and retired jack-of-all-trades who liked to spend Friday nights singing Jim Reeves songs and playing guitar at his local VFW, had invited me into his home so we could talk about what happened to him. "People around here know me for being smart, for knowing how to fix a lot of things," he told me the first time I met him, not long before showing me the paperwork that suggested he was unfit to father children. In 1948, when he was fourteen years old, Willis was taken from the state-run children's home where he lived to a nearby hospital. He remembered singing a country song to a nurse who held a mask over his face, counting backward, then waking up barely able to walk. Though it took a while for him to realize what had been done—no one talked to him about the surgery—he has lived most of his life with the knowledge that he will never have biological children.

By the time I met Willis, he'd become an advocate for compensation from our state's legislature, driving his 1982 Ford EXP to Raleigh to speak at hearings convened to consider how the state might make amends. He and other victims of the eugenics program thought that the government should recognize

these wrongs through memorials, education, and financial repa-
rations. Willis likened the payments to the financial compensation awarded to wrongfully convicted inmates. Though no
amount of money could make up for what North Carolina took
from him, he felt the state should put something on the line.

I was interested in the story of North Carolina's sterilization victims not because I had experienced anything like the
violence they suffered, but because the public and legislative response to their stories, and particularly their fight for financial
compensation, was dismissive in a way that I thought I recognized. *It was a long time ago,* some legislators claimed. Com-
menters on online stories about the victims wondered if perhaps
some people shouldn't be allowed to reproduce, unconsciously
echoing the dangerous and scientifically bankrupt ideas of the
first eugenicists. The refusal to recognize reproductive health
as vital, with lifelong consequences, had become familiar to me.

Few if any studies have been made about the psychological
damage of sterility, but there is evidence that infertility, as a
stressor, is equivalent to the experience of living with cancer,
HIV, or other chronic illnesses. "It's such an assault to your
identity," said Dr. Marni Rosner, a New York–based psychotherapist and the author of a lengthy study examining infertility
as a traumatic loss. "Physically, mentally, socially, spiritually."

Rosner's study focused on women whose backgrounds are
far different from those of victims of eugenics-based steriliza-
tions; they are comparatively wealthy and well connected, with
access to mental-health care and other support systems. But
the stories they told her about alienation and shame were
similar to the stories I heard from North Carolina's eugenics
victims. They describe feeling isolated from their churches,
especially on Mother's Day, when many congregations have
special recognition for mothers and expectant mothers. They
experience shame, depression, grief, envy, and difficulty communicating with spouses, family, and friends.

Rosner was the first in her field to fully explore the way infertility traumatically impacts almost every area of life, and was questioned about her use of the phrase *reproductive trauma* during her dissertation defense. "It's not concrete," she allowed. "The losses are hidden. But with reproductive trauma, the losses happen over and over again."

Compounding this sense of loss is the inability of many infertile people to talk about their experiences. As Rosner writes in her study, "There are no clear norms for grieving the loss of a dream." Fear of having one's loss diminished and the desire not to offend or upset those with children reinforce the silence that is a manifestation of what writer and grief counseling expert Kenneth Doka called "disenfranchised grief": "the grief that persons experience when they incur a loss that is not or cannot be openly acknowledged, publicly mourned, or socially supported."

It isn't surprising that sterilization victims have experienced social isolation, depression, trouble in their romantic relationships, and—perhaps most of all—disenfranchised grief. Because their inability to have children was not a consequence of biology but a decision made by another, they feel lifelong shame at being deemed "unfit." At the hearings held by North Carolina's task force to determine the method of compensation, several of the speakers were in tears as they told their stories. Some who suspected they were targeted and sterilized refused to go through the process of verification necessary to make them eligible for possible compensation. They didn't want to know the truth.

This made Willis's frank testimony and openness to journalists all the more courageous to me. At the Norlina VFW, where I met him another evening, he was friendly with the other musicians and the couples who'd come to dance, but I noticed that he stood slightly apart from them, drinking bottled water alone in the kitchen and stepping outside during breaks. Things might

have been different if he had had children of his own. He might
have had a lasting marriage, someone to take out on Friday
nights. His child, too, might have been a part of things. He told
me he still wondered if a daughter would have come hear to
him sing, if a son would have been someone he could have been
proud of.

I thought about him in Iceland, where we'd traveled to forget
about our childlessness. Forgetting wasn't possible in Reykjavík,
though, with the Christmas season well under way, schools on
recess, and large cartoon images of naughty Yule lads (a kind
of Christmas elf) projected onto downtown buildings. Even
the Icelandic naming tradition is a reminder of the primacy of
the parent-child relationship; surnames typically end in -*son* or
-*dottir* ("son" or "daughter").

"It stays on your mind," Willis had said, back in North
Carolina.

In Iceland, Richard and I bought Christmas ornaments and
booked a glacier tour; we smiled at toddlers in restaurants and
babies in strollers. It did.

There's another kind of courage among the childless, which
is not the determination to talk about why you couldn't have
children but why you chose not to. Especially for women, the
decision to remain childless or child-free is often seen as suspect or temporary. For years young women have complained, in
America and elsewhere, about the near impossibility of obtaining voluntary tubal ligations. Women in their twenties and even
thirties report encountering doctors who talk about their own
parenting experience, tell them they're too young, or suggest
that they just haven't met the right man yet.

"When [doctors have] talked about the fulfillment that children bring, I've explained that I already have a longer list of
things I want to do than I could possibly achieve in a lifetime,"
writes Holly Brockwell, who at twenty-nine had been refused a

tubal ligation four times by the U.K.'s National Health Service physicians. It made no sense, Brockwell claimed in an essay for the *Guardian,* that she was considered old enough to have children and take care of them—a permanent decision, after all— but not old enough to decide against reproducing: "It feels like a double standard: we'll agree that you know your own mind as long as your decisions align with ours."

In her story "A Magic of Bags," which I published in the online literary magazine *At Length,* the writer Mecca Jamilah Sullivan uses magical realism to evoke a character at odds with her Harlem community's expectations for young women. Ilana Randolph, a teenage girl "wide as a refrigerator" and with a fondness for colorful hair extensions, "was sure the body must have some better use," writes Mecca. "She dreamed instead of lodging herself under the world's skin, irritating it, making it itch." When a man at the check-cashing place (she was fourteen and cashing a check won in a High School Heroes essay contest) praised her "baby-bouncin thighs,"

Ilana stared at him until she could feel herself buzzing just below the gray hair on his left arm. It was a good feeling, and so she focused harder, maintaining eye contact as she handed over her check and ID. Staring for all those minutes wasn't easy, but it was gratifying—many times, she felt the need to blink, but she rallied and instead intensified her stare, thinking of nothing but the meat of the arm, and the heat of the itching. Then, as the man handed her the cash, just before she began to turn away, he raised his right hand, brought it to the arm, and scratched. It was glorious.

Since the publication of *Blue Talk and Love,* the collection in which Ilana appears, Mecca has heard about that character from a number of readers, many of them mothers, who write to her or speak up at readings. They're interested in the unusual ways Ilana exerts power and control, even over her own body. "It has a lot to do with [her] attitude toward mothering," Mecca told me in an email. "The character makes a choice not only not to have children, but also not to menstruate—that's how clear she is that reproduction in the most standard sense is not for her."

Mecca often wears colorful braids or twists in her own long hair and says that readers have also been curious about the possibility that her characters have autobiographical origins. "I usually joke that the characters are all very different people, although quite a few of them are big black girls with strange colors in their hair," she said. On a deeper level, she connects to her fictional characters' "investment in creating radical joy, against whatever odds."

"But as a writer and a woman and a queer person and a woman of color, I find a real value in acquainting myself with my wants and prioritizing my own desire," said Mecca, who is also a professor at UMass Amherst and regularly publishes essays and articles about politics, popular culture, and literature. "I don't desire kids right now. I desire lots of things, lots of forms of connection and intimacy and love, but that really isn't one of them. If that changes down the line, I'll figure it out. But for now, I want to live the life I desire."

I asked what she thought about the term *childless*—or *childfree*? Did either term appeal to her? "What about just *woman?*" she replied. "Even if I had a child, I think I would prefer to be known as a woman. Or a writer."

"As I've gotten older, I've also gotten braver about just saying, No, I never wanted children," the novelist and short-story writer Michelle Latiolais told me, also by email. "Used to be one said that and people looked at you as though you had said you enjoyed eating babies for lunch over-easy."

Michelle was my professor in graduate school and has been a mentor and role model to me since I met her, when I was twenty-three. I can distinctly remember watching her prepare for our first grad-school gathering on campus, deftly covering a folding table with a thick linen tablecloth and setting out fizzy lemonade and homemade shortbread. The charmless concrete courtyard where we gathered was suddenly beautiful, filled with golden afternoon light and the smell of eucalyptus. I wasn't sure how old she was then, and I don't know now. She was and is the most elegant, precise, generous teacher and writer I have ever known.

"I was just really never much interested, and I was working toward other things," she said. "I felt and I feel this even more strongly now that we have plenty of children in the world, and so, so many who need care and attention."

Michelle has nurtured countless younger people through her teaching, and she is a model for the teacher I want to be: principled and firm, but also the kind who introduces you to your favorite novel and invites the whole class to her house for a Mexican feast. "When people ask if I have children, I often say, yes, twelve or eighteen, the number of graduate students who are in the Programs in Writing at UC Irvine," she said. "They're really, really fascinating, compelling people, who aren't children, though I like feeding them."

Michelle's girlhood was different from mine. A complicated relationship with difficult parents also made her wary of adding to the world's unhappiness, the world's burden. She never babysat, and perhaps this contributed to a lack of interest in babies.

Though I had a happy childhood, I was afraid that my ambition as a writer, combined with and connected to my sometimes-difficult personality, could make it hard for me to become the mother I thought children deserved. Or else motherhood would make it impossible for me to be the writer I always imagined growing into. Tillie Olsen's descriptions of the writing life, during her twenty child-rearing, working years—"the simplest circumstances for creation did not exist"—were a warning to me, but also a consolation.

The writer and journalist Cat Warren told me about looking through her childhood stories and essays and realizing that they were full of independent and adventurous escape fantasies that were also tied to the life and skills she knew. Cat, who grew up in rural Oregon and was a caretaker to her paralyzed mother, wanted to move to New Zealand to become a nurse; she described her childhood short stories as "Laura Ingalls Wilder, with unicorns added."

For a long time she wanted nothing to do with motherhood or family life. She plotted her escape again in college, majoring in French so she could move to France post-graduation. There she decided to become a journalist. "I wanted to write about everything," she remembered. She dated and had relationships with men, but nothing that lasted; her life was about movement, adventure, and activism.

In her thirties, Cat went back to graduate school and felt the first pangs of baby fever. She told herself that if she became pregnant by accident, she'd have the child. She didn't get pregnant and at thirty-eight tried artificial insemination, which didn't result in a pregnancy. She got married, had a miscarriage, and got divorced. By then she'd become a professor of English at North Carolina State University, and her settled life had more room for a child. She began adoption proceedings with an agency that handled adoptions from Vietnam, completed a home study and psychological evaluation, called on friends to write letters of recommendation. Imagining and preparing for this new life, she bought a house in a district with an excellent, diverse elementary school.

Then she met David Auerbach, a tall, Bronx-born baker of bread and professor of philosophy, and the two fell in love. A few months later she was diagnosed with breast cancer.

"'What do we do?'" Cat remembered asking herself and

asking David. She had not been matched but was already deep into the adoption process. She still very much wanted a child. "Whatever I wanted, David would have gone along with it."

Though Cat kept the file folder of adoption paperwork—it's hard to let go of a dream—she decided that continuing with the adoption, considering her uncertain health, was not responsible. "None of the equations worked to bring a child into our lives," she said.

After two surgeries and radiation, Cat's cancer went into remission, and she has had no recurrences. She and David married in 2001; they live in Durham in a cohousing community David founded. All of the individually owned houses face a central courtyard planted with fruit trees and stocked with beehives, and they are surrounded by neighbors with children. In 2013, Cat published the bestselling *What the Dog Knows,* an intensely researched book inspired by her experience training a spirited German shepherd to do search-and-rescue work, which brought more people, including children, into her life as well.

"I wouldn't say David and I are childless," Cat told me. "And *child-free* sounds like a PR riff . . . I don't relate to either term."

In addition to family and neighbors, Cat and David have been especially close to Reginald, the autistic son of a close friend who died of cancer several years ago. As a child Reginald adored her two German shepherds, Solo and Zev, and Cat once watched him tell a group of tough boys in a park, "This is Zev, my dog." She showed me how he placed his hand lightly on Zev's head and raised his own in an expression of pride and belonging.

In some ways Cat decided not to have children, and in some ways life decided for her. "It would be wrong to say I don't have regrets," she said. She described a familiar melancholy that sometimes descends on Sundays. "I would have, given all my druthers, liked to be surrounded a little more."

Michelle doesn't have regrets but also had a time when she surrendered to what-might-be, giving up on birth control and deciding, with her husband, Paul, that they would have the child if she became pregnant. "We would never have gotten married if I'd had medical coverage, but at the time, I didn't and needed it, and so we got married," Michelle said. "What surprised and angered both Paul and me after we did was that people now felt completely entitled to ask us very personal questions. Or to say to us, 'You got married because you're pregnant, right?' We were really stunned by this and actually even joked about getting divorced so that we could say, 'We're getting divorced because Michelle's pregnant' so they could really have something to talk about!"

The writer Elizabeth Tallent once told Michelle that if she'd had children, she wouldn't pay so much attention to them—I imagine Tallent meant in her writing, which often considers the intelligence and force of both women and children, and also in the classroom. "I am not sure I'd be as open to students as I hope I am if I had children of my own," Michelle allowed. "So, 'child-free' allows me to be better at something than I would perhaps be if kindered."

I thought of my favorite teachers across my whole educational experience: the ones who invited me for tea or let me monopolize their office hours, or who took care of me in elementary school when my brother was hospitalized for asthma. With the exception of a beloved high school English teacher, they were all childless. Or child-free. Or unkindered.

"I love her," my friend told me, "because she doesn't worry about being alone." We were sitting on a grassy hillside in Raleigh, and Neko Case was singing, *That echo chorus lied to me with its / "Hold on, hold on, hold on, hold on."* Like Case, my friend is single, in her forties, and childless. It was the second time we'd seen her perform together—the first time, two years earlier, I'd had a similar thought about the singer: she has no children, but look at her life.

It seems wrong to burden our teachers and artists with the responsibility of mothering, or even modeling a life that looks more like our own and less like our mothers'. This is a narrow and selfish view of their talents and gifts, one that willfully ignores the complex and private histories that shaped the lives we emulate.

And yet I'm grateful, greedy, for every kind of model. For Cat, who is researching a new book about climate change and farming, and who told me that she suspected we all wind up at about the same place, happiness-wise. For Michelle, with her fierce conviction that we owe all children an education, health care, and exposure to arts and culture. For Mecca, who creates impressive female characters who battle convention. And for Willis, who remained a devoted son and uncle and became a determined and effective advocate for justice, contributing to the first movement that secured compensation for eugenics victims in America. Cat and Willis, who both wanted children, embody what Rosner describes as "post-traumatic growth"—the ability to expand one's identity beyond a life crisis, creating positive change in its aftermath.

Richard and I didn't see the northern lights in Iceland; it was too cloudy. We took a four-wheel-drive tour that hit the usual sights: Þingvellir National Park, the waterfall at Gullfoss, Geysir. In the early afternoon our guide and driver, a burly man named Birgir, took us and another couple to the base of Langjökull, the second-largest ice cap in Iceland. At its greatest height Langjökull is more than four thousand feet above sea level, and we had to stop next to a sign that read "Ófært! Impassable" and deflate the tires before making the ascent. Birgir put Russian techno on the stereo and cranked it, steering the superjeep with one hand along the rutted road. We finally stopped at a snowmobile camp, and Richard and I got out to hike in deep snow.

It was the shortest day of the year, the sky already darkening. I'd imagined hiking on actual ice, with crampons fastened over our boots. Instead we trekked across the tundra, a wide, featureless expanse that evoked the endlessness of dreamspace. It was cold, and too windy to hear each other or the distant snowmobilers, by now racing across the glacier. We moved more slowly, trudging toward a rock that looked from far away like a small mountain. It took a long time to reach the rock, and we took turns standing on it and striking heroic poses. Everything—land and sky, snow and clouds—began merging into the gray-blue dusk. We scratched our initials in the snow, as we had in the sand at the beach last Christmas, the most ephemeral of gestures. R + B.

There have been times in my life when what felt like an unbearably strong desire to be different than I am has finally subsided into something like peace or acceptance. Before I published my first book, I was working long hours at a KIPP charter school in D.C. My agent then, who I hoped would help me find a home for the collection, didn't return my emails, and all my writing and submission time was given over to tasks that felt more urgent: lesson planning, grading, and managing paperwork related to KIPP's draconian method of student discipline. This was also the year I started trying to get pregnant.

Richard, who worked longer hours than I did, understood my frustration and my desire. We both wanted our lives to be different than they were—wanted more time together and for writing, wanted a family, wanted to move back to our house in North Carolina. That winter, without telling me, he printed and sent my collection of stories to a contest, and it won. I can still remember the elation and disbelief I felt talking to the poet Michael Collier, who called on the last day of my school's spring break to tell me the book would be published.

When I relate that story to other writers, I use it to emphasize two things: first, how important it is to have people in your life who believe in you, but also how crucial it is to believe in and stick by your own work. I didn't do that, I tell people—though Richard's act was the most generous and unexpected gift I've ever been given, I should have been a better advocate for my own work. I should have severed ties with an agent who wasn't interested in representing the work I wanted to write, should have mailed my book to the contest myself.

But there is something harder to convey in this story, something that I think is also instructive. That winter I remember stepping through our front door after an eleven- or twelve-hour workday, looking longingly at my unused writing desk, and thinking, *Even if the last book doesn't sell* (it didn't), *and even if this book goes nowhere too, I'll write another one. I'll keep going.* I felt an enormous and sudden relief knowing that, no matter what happened, I'd find a way to keep writing.

Something similar happened around the time Richard and I went to Iceland. I hadn't given up on my treatment, but I finally understood that, even if we were unsuccessful this time, and the next, and the time after that, we'd be okay. I'd of course said this before—*We'll be okay* was almost a mantra—but now I believed the words I so often uttered. It wasn't going to Iceland and standing on a glacier that helped me, but an accumulation of experiences: getting to know Willis, who was so open and courageous; going month after month to our support group, where we felt understood; living my life as a writer, a daughter, a wife.

This sense of peace and acceptance feels like wisdom, but I think it's nature: the body and mind letting go, making room for change. However the feeling originates, I've learned to welcome it. Richard and I flew home from Iceland at dusk on Christmas Eve. The day was longer than the one before, if only by a minute or two, and for a long time our westward-flying plane tracked the sunset. I watched its blazing, then fading, colors and thought about what was next.

The Whole House

...

The well diggers arrived on a windy late-January morning, too unseasonably warm to ask them, as I joked with my father that I would, about the relative coldness of their asses. Besides, it isn't done that way anymore—no shovels or crouching down or even actual digging. Their three large trucks barely made it up our steep gravel driveway. One truck carried water to cool the drill and flush the well of debris; one hauled the twenty-foot drill bits that would bore into the earth; and one held the rig, which supported and powered the drilling. Before they could even position the rig above our well, which we had hired them to dig deeper, they had to cut down a poplar tree and a sweet-gum tree and some hollies. The trees were felled, sectioned, and rolled over the hill in minutes, while I watched, wincing, from the kitchen window. *It's okay,* I told myself. *We have plenty of trees but not enough water.*

I'd known this day was coming ever since Richard and I bought our house more than six years ago and noticed the black coil of tubing that once carried water from our neighbor's house to ours, back when they were both rental properties. "You know how renters are," Bill Spiegel said when we asked about the tubing. Back in 1975, the year before Richard and I were born, Bill built the cabin entirely of handmade and salvaged materials, designing its footprint and post-and-beam construction around the existing trees and steep grade of the land. When he couldn't salvage windows large enough to accommodate the passive solar design and views he wanted, he had glass cut and framed it himself. The cedar posts supporting the roof and rafters were collected from the property; they rest on rocks Bill dug up and buried. Everything about the house is seventies-era DIY. "Bill did all this," our plumber said dismissively, "when he was vibing on life."

On the day we first saw the house, Bill pointed out the layout's good feng shui; the large, south-facing windows; the old claw-foot tub and beauty-shop sink he'd restored. By the time we walked all five acres and visited the property's shared easement to the Haw River, we decided not to worry too much about the ominous tubing or the mysterious presence of two wells instead of one. After moving in, we quickly found that Bill was right— there was something ineffable that made the house feel bigger than its eight hundred square feet. We loved that we didn't have to hang curtains in any of the windows, that we could sleep with the French doors to the screen porch wide open in the spring and summertime, listening to the night song of crickets and cicadas and owls.

We figured we would make do with whatever water our two low-producing wells provided, and we put off calling well drillers as long as we could. We grew accustomed to the inconvenience: strategically choosing the best time to do laundry, jumping out of a weak shower and streaking across the driveway to switch tanks, washing dishes with just a trickle of water. In a way, the meagerness of our wells had a positive effect, reminding us to conserve, to be mindful of at least that one limited resource, which we monitored via a gauge in our garage. I was highly attuned to the condition of both wells, even though I couldn't see what was inside them, and also constantly afraid of running out of water. But when is it ever a good time to spend thousands of dollars on something with uncertain results? Though Richard and I both have degrees in fine arts, we thought the answer was never.

"There's no guarantee," Mr. Maness told me cheerfully, once the rig was already drilling. W. W. Maness and Sons hold Chatham County's drilling permit number 58, a sign of how long they've been doing business here. It's true, there is no guarantee, no way to know whether drilling any well a few hundred feet deeper will yield more water or what they call a dry hole. In the hilly and rocky land around our property, unlucky farmers and landowners have been known to drill one after another. Even the most skeptical will enlist dousers, who "witch" the land with a forked stick to determine the best spot for drilling. *Why not?* they figure. Dousers work for a nominal fee—some old-timers won't accept payment at all—and everyone has a neighbor or friend with a high-producing well somebody witched.

We were down two hundred feet already, and there was no more water—"not a drop," Mr. Maness said. At ten dollars a foot, and an eight-hundred-dollar setup fee to position their truck over our existing well, we were already in it for close to three grand. Work slowed while the men hoisted a new drill bit onto the rig, then lowered it into the hole. I stood and watched the heavy rod slowly disappear, while behind the rig, wastewater and rock fragments spewed into the trees. I tried not to think about the money.

"We checked their well tag, and they got twenty gallons a minute at six forty," Mr. Maness told me, pointing up the hill at my other neighbors' well. I knew that and was prepared to go that deep, though I also knew that my neighbors didn't hit anything before they got to 640.

"You think the water's just that far down?" I asked, picturing an aquifer, blue and level, as in a textbook.

Mr. Maness shrugged. *It's more like veins,* he told me, tracing a twisted pattern in the air with his hand. But he hoped we'd hit water before too long.

I wished I could ask my neighbors about the waiting, if they felt like giving up at 500 feet, or at 550 or 600, but two years ago they had twins, and they moved to town.

Back inside the house I returned to my other preoccupation, also fraught with worries about money and uncertainty. I'd spent the past two days calling pharmacies to find the best price on medication to suppress, then stimulate, my ovaries for my first cycle of in vitro fertilization.

It took us so long to make this decision—more than two years since we first met our reproductive endocrinologist—that Dr. Young's office had moved from a nearby university hospital to a new office complex in the Raleigh suburbs. But I still had notes from meetings with him scattered throughout a pocket-sized notebook, and I could distinctly remember our first appointment, when he said, "I'm ninety percent sure I can get you pregnant with IVF." IVF seemed a long way away then—there were other, less expensive treatments to try first—and I did not write his prediction down, so I had only my memory that he said it, and the way Richard and I both bristled at the idea that a *doctor* would get me pregnant.

The presence of medicine in something so deeply personal, so long hoped for, so much a part of how we envision ourselves, is perhaps the rudest awakening within the experience of assisted reproduction. No one imagines that she will need to be tested, medicated, and injected before conceiving a child, that her eggs will have to be retrieved and combined in a laboratory with her partner's sperm before being transferred back to her body. Like water, our bodies and their generative capacity are something most of us take for granted.

So we tried the other, less invasive methods first: tried oral medication, tried intrauterine insemination and acupuncture and natural-cycle timing and taking a break from actively trying. In July 2012, after all those methods failed, we visited our doc-

tor again, and I took notes about a possible IVF cycle. Among
my pencil scribbles were terse phrases expressing my incomplete understanding of what it would be like: "Moderate level
of meds" and "Morning ultrasound, five times" and "six-week
process" and "two weeks really busy." I drew a line under those
notes, then wrote "appx. $13,000 including meds, one try."

As with our upper well, which had been failing since the
summer, I knew that our time was running out. At thirty-six,
I was already past the age at which fertility precipitously declines. I had accommodated my life to childlessness in as many
ways as I accommodated a scarcity of water. But still it felt as
though we were missing something essential. Because having
a child was something I'd always taken for granted, it was difficult to imagine or understand my life without that experience.
Why had I bothered to store away all this information about raising children? Why had I saved all of these picture books, and
bought this house in the country, and married this man? Why
had I imagined myself as a mother, and Richard as a father?

So we did it—we scheduled and took our blood tests right before our trip to Iceland, and we paid the money a few days after
we returned, more than I'd ever paid at one time for anything
in my life. We watched YouTube videos on how to inject Lupron
into the upper thigh, how to mix the Follistim and Menopur into
a single dose before injecting it into a pinch of stomach fat.

Obtaining the Lupron, the Follistim, and the Menopur was
another matter. The specialty mail-order pharmacy that miraculously accepted my insurance was slow and uncertain. They
could not tell me when it would ship, only that I had to be patient. No one I spoke to knew how to pronounce the medicine I
was ordering, or what it was for (maybe this is why it was covered by insurance), and they did not seem to understand that
the schedule my nurse emailed me required me to begin my
medicine on a certain (fast approaching) day.

I called the number for the second time that morning, hoping the customer service agents would be able to hear me over the low drone of drilling that shook our small house.

The prerecorded message reminded me that things could be worse. "If you are an oncology patient, please press two. For Avonex patients, please press three. For MS patients who are not taking Avonex, please press four. If you are a hepatitis patient, please press five." I pressed seven, for "all other patients," and tried to think about the ways that I was lucky.

But once on the phone with a representative, I found myself channeling the will of a patient ordering something life sustaining. "I need this medicine," I told the woman who slowly read through my order, spelling out *Leuprolide* rather than trying to pronounce it. "I have to have it by Wednesday."

"I'll mark it Urgent," she told me, without promising anything.

I told her I'd call back in a few hours.

I hung up and went outside with my camera, snapping photos of the trucks, the tall rig, the pale mud coating nearby trees: documentation of the expense, the effort. Then I stood near the rig, my hands cupped over my ears. Mr. Maness noticed me and walked over with an apologetic look. We were down to six hundred feet, without any more water to show for it. I tried to picture six hundred feet vertical and found that I could not.

They had used all the drill bits that they brought and would have to come back tomorrow with more. "Rock's changing," he told me, describing how it was now darker and softer. That I could picture: rock crumbling like clay, giving over to water. "That could be a good sign. But we won't go more than a couple hundred more feet. After that, we'll have to stop."

Bill Spiegel still calls our house the hippie house when introducing us to neighbors; the label is actually listed on the plat. Back when he first built it, the structure was a single thirty-two-by-sixteen-foot room. He fed his woodstove with trees felled on the property, cooked meals on a two-burner hot plate powered by temporary service from the electric company—essentially an outlet wired to a post in the yard—and slept in a loft above the bathroom, which had the claw-foot tub and sink that first charmed us but no toilet and no door. He used an outhouse or peed in the yard for five years, until he dated a woman who got so fed up with his version of country living that she finally roped a bartered toilet to the back of his Volkswagen Bug while he was at work at Glaxo, a pharmaceutical company in Raleigh. "The company photographer took a picture of it," he told me. He drove the toilet home and installed it, and the girlfriend stayed for a few more years.

He doesn't live that way anymore—he has a three-thousand-square-foot house on ten acres across the road, another place he built on the river, and an apartment in a LEED-certified building in Chapel Hill. Still, the ethos of the back-to-the-land movement that drew Bill and others like him to Chatham County in the 1970s is evident all around us, not so much in the now-older (and considerably wealthier) hippies who are our neighbors but in the deed to our house and land, which carry with them a restrictive covenant designed to resist the suburban values Bill and his fellow homesteaders were fleeing. Just a few miles down the road, new developments with names like Chapel Ridge and Laurel Estates promise a different kind of life, their hulking brick-faced houses ("From the $370s," read the signs) fed by massive water towers and barely shaded by tall, widely spaced pines. No one in our community can build closer than seventy-five feet to the property line; we can't put up halogen or sodium vapor lighting or build a McMansion. We can't cut down more than 50 percent of the trees on our lots or divide them into smaller parcels (all lots are five or more acres). And we can't have a whole passel of kids unless we want to buy more land—written into the covenant is the restriction that you must have one acre of land for each member of the household.

I like to picture each lot subdivided by imaginary lines, our neighbors standing out in the woods on their acre-or-more portions, arms spread wide as in a giant game of hippie four square. Richard says there's no way this rule is legally enforceable, but recently a real estate deal fell through when a family of six wanted to buy a five-acre lot. The sellers' agent drove all around with a proposal exempting the family from the covenant; we debated whether we'd sign (Richard was for the exemption; I was against), but it didn't matter in the end. No one else would sign it, and the family bought somewhere else.

The early to mid-1970s, just before Bill and his fellow homesteaders drafted their "one person per acre" covenant, is the one period in American history when having children—as many as you could afford to look after—slipped from favor. Cultural resistance to pronatalist ideology took many forms. Feminists decried the suffocation of marriage and motherhood, and proponents of child-free living began asserting the perks of life without kids: more time for romance, for travel and art and self-actualization. More money, better sex. "Take your pick," wrote Ellen Peck in her quaintly sexist 1971 book, *The Baby Trap,* which proposed child-free living as the best way to stay attractive and keep your man. "Housework and children—or the glamour, involvement and excitement of a free life." But perhaps most compelling, to men and women who wanted to preserve every possible tree and shield the night sky from the glare of useless lampposts, was the argument Paul Ehrlich made in *The Population Bomb:* there were too many of us already.

By the early 1970s, Ehrlich's bestselling book had grown into a full-blown movement: ZPG, or Zero Population Growth, an organization with chapters in thirty states. Ehrlich saw population growth as a "cancer" that could no longer be treated but had to be excised before mankind bred itself to extinction. "The mother of the year should be a sterilized woman with two adopted children," he was fond of telling the audiences greeting him at college campuses around the country. If that sounded unappealing, he had an easy-to-remember fallback plan: "Stop at Two."

It appeared to be working: by 1975, the year Bill built our house and envisioned a covenant restricting its occupants, the American fertility rate had fallen from 3.4 children per woman to 1.8 children, producing an overall population decline of one percent per year. One point eight children: you can picture them in a yurt or a tiny "hippie house" like ours. Or no children—in the copies of *Shelter* and *Woodstock Handmade Houses* Richard has collected from thrift stores around town, the yurts, cabins, and shacks are empty, too neat to be the homes of children. Flipping through the brownish photographs, I see looms and easels and woodworking stations but no cribs or toys.

Stopping at two implies replacement, equilibrium. Zero population growth: there is something elegant about that math. In my support group, most people said they'd be satisfied—delighted, even—with one, or with a child they could be sure of adopting as an infant. But no one wanted to make up for the hyper-fertile: even Ehrlich fathered a child before his vasectomy.

That night I presented the options to Richard as Mr. Maness explained them to me: stop drilling and limp along, keep drilling and hope to hit more water, drill a new well somewhere else, or restore the well we had. I'd already calculated the price of each option and its relative damage to our savings. Well restoration, which involved forcing hundreds of gallons of pressurized water into low-producing wells, would easily cost $5,000, but so would drilling a new well. Nothing could guarantee more water.

I grew up in a hundred-year-old log cabin and was familiar with the many ways a house and its property can turn on you: fallen trees, frozen pipes, wells swamped with greenish storm water. Richard grew up in the suburbs of D.C., and I worried, when we bought this house, that he might be put off by its inconveniences. As a couple, we had lived only in cities, and we'd moved almost every year to a new apartment, a new neighborhood. We appreciated the convenience of calling the landlord when something broke or needed to be serviced, and the proximity of restaurants, music, shops. The house we bought—this house—is ten miles from the nearest gas station. Our covenant restricting outdoor lights makes nights pitch-black except for the stars, and back when we moved in, I wondered, what if Richard freaks out, like my New York–born grandmother, who drew all the never-used, army-green shades in our cabin and taped them down with masking tape?

But the house, the life we live here, has changed him. He appreciates the privacy and the chance to learn skills—plumbing, chainsawing, driveway maintenance—that were previously unnecessary. He's stocked our bookshelves with books on home repair and using salvaged materials *(Electrical Basics, How to Build Furniture without Tools)*, and with those hand-built-housing manuals from the 1970s. Lately he'd become interested in emergency preparedness, a response I suspected was as related to the isolation of our personal circumstances as it was to the increased frequency of powerful storms and long droughts.

"I don't know what we'll do if they don't hit water," I told him, scrolling through a table of well-restoration data I found online. This was my real fear, both for the well and for IVF—that our efforts would not work, and, resources depleted, we would have to figure out something else.

Richard was calm, his mind bent not to subtraction but to addition. "It'll be okay," he told me. He could figure out how to earn the extra money we needed, he said. I was struck by how much, in his calm material determination, he reminded me of my own father, and also by how readily we were falling into traditional gender roles, as if by conforming we might have a better chance of getting what we wanted. He gathered the resources; I managed them while agitating for more. An old story.

I often make Richard promise me things he has no ability to predict, but I knew better than to do that now. Instead I told him about the pharmacy phone calls and my suspicion that no one I knew could understand the vocabulary of both dilemmas— gallons per minute in a deep rock well, follicle suppression and stimulation through injectable medications (though perhaps our neighbors knew something of both, it occurred to me later). In some ways our goals felt ridiculously modest—one baby, a slightly bigger house, enough water to wash clothes and shower without worrying—and that was alienating too. "A gallon a minute," I said. "I'd settle for that." I was sure we could function on a gallon a minute.

I sometimes had nightmares involving broken eggs with yolks and shells, but lately those had been replaced by pleasant dreams about babies. I dreamed of the heft of their little torsos, the sweet smell of their heads, their laughing faces. None of them looked especially like me or Richard, and I wasn't even aware, in my dreams, that they were ours.

But that was what I was thinking about the next morning when I woke up: babies. Then I remembered the well-drilling rig still parked expensively up my hill, and the uncertainty.

Richard stayed home in case we didn't hit water, so we could decide together whether to give up or tell them to drill in a different spot. The men started early. By now I could tell by sound alone when they were drilling and when the truck was idling. I sat on the sofa and tried to work while Richard stood at the window and watched. "Something's changing," he said after a while. "There's more water."

I got up and looked at the place where the rig blew waste and exhaust into the woods. "It always looks like that," I said. "It looked like that yesterday."

But a few minutes later, Richard reported that the men were mucking around with shovels and a scoop cut from a plastic gallon jug. They were fitting a new length of PVC onto the exhaust pipe and digging a trench in the grayish sludge that had once been solid rock. We were still guessing at what it could mean when Mr. Maness came to the door.

"You'll be okay now," he said. "You've got five gallons a minute."

We high-fived; we did a dance of happiness. Five gallons a minute would be enough for us, and even enough for a family. I stepped onto the damp porch in my socks and watched Mr. Maness make his way back to the rig, where he had still more to do: additional drilling to get beneath the vein, then extracting the thirty-four sections of drill bits that had finally, far below, found water. It could have easily gone the other way. We have some neighbors with deep, dry wells and others who could supply an entire farm with water. We wound up in the middle, but we never intended to start a farm.

"That'll be plenty," Mr. Maness reassured us again, before he and his crew left in their three trucks. "Plenty for the whole house."

Takeover

· · ·

In February our tap water still smelled of chlorine tablets disinfecting the well we drilled the month before, giving our tiny house the damp, close feel of an indoor public pool. I was running load after load of white laundry, trying to flush out the chemicals, when the UPS driver arrived with my first shipment of IVF medication. I signed for the three large cardboard boxes, marked PERISHABLE OPEN UPON RECEIPT. They were surprisingly light, like props, and I waved off the driver's offer of help and carried them inside.

After the truck was gone, I sliced open each box to find rounded Styrofoam coolers and frozen gel packs protecting my cartons of Lupron, Follistim, and Menopur. I set the medicine, the syringes, the sharps container, and the alcohol swabs on my kitchen table: more shots than my body had ever received, more medicine than I had ever taken. I photographed the eleven cartons of drugs, the three sizes of needles, the pages-long lists of instructions and precautions; then I put them all away where I wouldn't have to see them.

The phrase my doctor uses to describe the way IVF works is *take over*—*We'll take over your whole cycle,* he told me enthusiastically. As in, *Don't worry about your short luteal phase, your thin uterine lining, or predicting when you might ovulate. Your body*

will not be trusted to perform any of its biological tasks. We will do
it all for you. To you.

The first means of this takeover is often Lupron, a drug prescribed to treat early-onset puberty, prostate cancer, and endometriosis and to delay puberty in children who might be transgender. In IVF, Lupron has a primarily suppressive effect; those new to IVF protocols are often surprised to see that they will first take birth control pills, then Lupron and birth control simultaneously. They'll wait to get their periods, continue taking Lupron, then add a gonadotropin, or follicle-stimulating hormone, while easing off the dosage of Lupron. Lupron shuts off portions of the pituitary gland, tricking the body into thinking it is menopausal; fertility doctors use it to prevent ovarian cysts from forming, to time the onset of menstruation, and to suppress the body's natural tendency to promote the development of a single follicle. IVF's goal is many follicles, many eggs, and Lupron makes that possible. Like a lot of medications used in reproductive endocrinology, it's prescribed off label.

I googled "dangers of Lupron" and found personal stories posted to message boards, court cases and testimonials on lupronvictimshub.com, advertisements from attorneys, and a detailed (and convincing) overview of the risks from National Women's Health Network, a feminist health-care lobbying group. According to an article by Susan K. Flinn, editor of the Women's Health Activist newsletter, "there have been no prospective or clinical studies on Lupron's safety for ART patients." Flinn notes that it causes birth defects and is categorized by OSHA as a hazardous drug; OSHA advises health-care workers to don protective gloves while handling Lupron, and those intending to get pregnant or father a child to avoid it entirely. Flinn sprinkles her article with posts from distraught patients, including this one, collected from lupronvictimshub.com:

I have been to a total of 17 doctors since taking Lupron with many different diagnoses and there doesn't seem to be an end in sight. I don't know why we can't seem to get someone in the medical field to look into the on-going side effects of this drug. There is something definitely wrong with a drug when you go from being perfectly healthy to having all kinds of medical problems and you know that in your heart it started while on Lupron. I do know that I am not alone. I used to think I was but I have personally spoken to people that have [taken] Lupron and they are experiencing the same problems.

It's hard to know, in an ART cycle, exactly which drug is causing which side effects, but I'd heard plenty of complaints about Lupron—hot flashes, tearfulness, anxiety. Possible long-term side effects of prolonged Lupron therapy—the kind prescribed for severe endometriosis and uterine fibroids—include bone-density loss, debilitating headaches, chronic generalized pain, depression, immune system disorders, and paralysis. Takeda Abbott Pharmaceuticals, the drug company that manufactures Lupron, paid $875 million in 2001 to settle a claim that it promoted Lupron to doctors through illegal kickbacks and Medicare fraud. I found reports online that the FDA has received between twelve thousand and twenty-two thousand reports of adverse events linked to Lupron, including hundreds of deaths.

In the conventional IVF cycle our doctor recommended, I'd inject this drug for two weeks. It would have been possible to limit my exposure either with a natural-cycle IVF, which would harvest the single egg my body might naturally produce, or with something called an antagonist protocol, which supplants Lupron with an antagonist such as Ganirelix. Our doctor told me that Lupron down-regulation, in which Lupron is prescribed to control the onset of menstruation and suppress initial follicle development, had the best success rates for someone in my circumstances. All of our choices so far (except waiting) had been carefully made to maximize our chances—at Dr. Young's suggestion, we even skipped the first cohort of IVF patients to be treated in our clinic's new laboratory, just in case there were kinks to be worked out.

By the time I received my six-week calendar of medication from the clinic, my fear had already shifted, a common experience among those moving up the fertility-treatment ladder. A friend who became pregnant after years of treatment by three different reproductive endocrinologists put it this way: "In the beginning I definitely worried about the long term effects of the hormonal drugs on my health, yet as I got further along, I cared less about the consequences on myself. I remember thinking that I would *never* do IVF or take the heavy duty drugs."

I thought the same thing. But the IVF cycle, so complicated and demanding, replaces fear for your own body with anxiety over its production, and you suddenly wonder, *Will it be enough?* My friend, a scientist and former Peace Corps volunteer, got accepted into a study at one of the premier "natural cycle" IVF clinics in the country—the same clinic that gave Martha Stewart her first grandchild—and traveled to New York to participate. The study was evaluating the difference between "mini" IVF, which calls for minimal injectable medication, and conventional IVF, which requires between thirty and fifty injections. Doctors using mini IVF collect one or two eggs per cycle, while conventional methods could produce twenty or more. The protocols were randomly assigned, and my friend drew the conventional one: lots of those expensive shots she once dreaded. But she was relieved, even after months of research about the benefits of mini IVF: less stress on her ovaries, no risk of ovarian hyperstimulation, potentially healthier eggs. When it came time to begin the cycle, she wanted the greatest number of eggs, the best chance of success.

. . .

For most of human history, doctors knew less about human reproduction than what today's average middle-schooler learns in health class. The presence of eggs, or ova, was not confirmed until 1827; it took another sixteen years for scientists to discover that sperm must fertilize an egg for conception to take place. Though folk remedies for infertility had been practiced for thousands of years, the Western medical establishment would bumble along for decades before finding promising treatments. Marion Sims, a surgeon-gynecologist working in the mid-nineteenth century, assumed the problem was one of access: to help the sperm better find their target, he widened his patients' cervixes with a terrifying-looking speculum and completed an early study of artificial insemination, which he called "ethereal copulation." Out of fifty-five attempts with six couples, he reported only one success, possibly because he believed that ovulation occurred during menstruation. Others looked for infertility's causes—Harvard professor of medicine Edward Clarke suggested in 1873 that too much education gave women "monstrous brains and puny bodies," injuring their reproductive organs. Men, it was commonly believed, became infertile through sex with prostitutes (this was likely true for some).

Though the early twentieth century brought discoveries of important sex hormones and fertility tests, patients had to wait until the late 1950s for promising but risky hormonal treatments, using medication sourced from the pituitary glands of cadavers and the urine of post-menopausal women. Carl Gemzell, the Swedish doctor who pioneered the use of gonadotropin to stimulate egg production in acyclic women, nearly ended his research after one of his patients gave birth prematurely to six babies, who all died. "I felt I hadn't the right to let even one more patient run the terrible risk of having so many babies," Gemzell told the *Australian Women's Weekly* in 1966. By then Gemzell's protocol had spread to clinics in seven different countries. "To do what I had done—to be the instrument of making a woman bear the agony of giving birth to six children at once was a frightful thing to do," he said. Gemzell changed his mind soon after, when four of his patients each gave birth to a single, healthy child. Those babies, he said, renewed his hope and confidence: "The joy on the faces of their mothers, the happiness of the fathers—oh, it was wonderful to see." Gemzell and the other doctors using his protocol of injectable gonadotropin attempted to use the lowest effective dose, but it was impossible to predict the outcome of each cycle. Some patients bore healthy singletons, while others faced traumatic births of up to seven babies. Infertile couples were willing to risk treatment, perhaps imagining a crowded nursery rather than the reality of long hospital stays and painful deaths. "Four, five, even six babies—it was a gamble we decided to take," a Swedish housewife told the same magazine. "We wanted a child so very much." Years later, some of Gemzell's patients died from Creutzfeldt-Jacob disease, apparently transmitted by the cadavers he used to source gonadotropin.

Though their treatment was risky and clumsy by today's standards, Gemzell's patients were among the first to experience the takeover of their reproductive systems, and the therapy he developed—injectable gonadotropin—is still used worldwide by reproductive endocrinologists. It's difficult to imagine what women considering or experiencing treatment might have thought—in the pre-Internet era, there were no message boards on which to share fears or hard-won research, and stories in the press, though they reported the deaths of sextuplets and septuplets, often gave voice only to happy mothers. *Five babies. How lucky!* an infertile woman may have thought, gazing at a photograph of a beaming, attractive mother of adorable quints.

Reproductive medicine has a long history of absent or incomplete patient understanding. The first recorded artificial insemination by a donor was performed in 1884 on a wealthy Philadelphia woman who happened to be anesthetized—and who would never know that her son's biological father was a handsome young medical student and not her own (gonorrheal) husband. Lesley Brown, a British factory worker and the first IVF patient to give birth, had no idea she was a pioneer. "I don't remember Mr. Steptoe saying his method of producing babies had ever worked, and I certainly didn't ask. I just imagined that hundreds of children had already been born through being conceived outside their mothers' wombs," she wrote in a 1979 memoir coauthored with her husband.

Unlike Gemzell's patients, and unlike most IVF recipients today, Brown's treatment was accomplished surgically, without medication to stimulate ovarian production. Her doctor, Patrick Steptoe, referred to it as an "implant," and the process sounded so simple to Brown that she "wouldn't have believed it if Mr. Steptoe had told me straight out that, after years of trying, no one had ever had a baby from an implant." But it had been years—more than twenty since scientist Robert Edwards began studying and conducting experiments on mouse, rat, hamster, sheep, cow, rhesus monkey, and human oocytes, and almost ten since he began working with Steptoe on the oocytes of volunteer patients. In 1977, the year she unwittingly made history, Brown was twenty-nine years old; blocked fallopian tubes had left her barren and depressed over her inability to conceive, but also the perfect candidate for Steptoe and Edwards's trial.

The two doctors had for a time administered gonadotropin to their infertile patients, producing mild ovarian stimulation and multiple egg-bearing follicles. Steptoe collected the oocytes through the delicate laparoscopic technique he developed in his gynecological practice. Edwards fertilized the mature eggs and grew them in various media; his descriptions of the resulting embryos, in an essay for *Nature Medicine* written decades later, still sound breathlessly pleased. "Most had normal nuclei, even-sized blastomeres and approximately diploid chromosomes, developed to a strict timetable, compacted excellently, secreted blastocoelic fluid, and were obviously vibrant as blastocysts with 100 or more nuclei and many mitoses on day 5. Some blastocysts grew to 9 days, their expanding embryonic discs stuffed full of embryonic stem cells!" But once they began transferring the embryos back to their mothers, in 1972, Steptoe and Edwards began to see problems related to their patients' hormonal treatment. They could fertilize mature eggs, watch as they developed into beautiful embryos, and transfer them back at just the right moment, but they could not control what happened next, within the woman's uterus.

"Something must be fundamentally flawed with a reproductive system that allows only 20% of embryos to implant, even in younger couples," Edwards complained near the end of his life. Back in the 1970s, the naturally low human implantation rate was compounded in clinical trials by the ovarian-stimulating medicine given to Steptoe's patients. This medication thinned the uterine lining or otherwise created short luteal phases, and some patients menstruated five to six days after ovulation. Not one was pregnant. Steptoe and Edwards experimented with different medications and techniques, including oocyte recovery with tubal insemination, but finally settled on natural cycle as the best way to establish IVF as a legitimate treatment of infertility.

Brown did not require hormonal treatment; she produced healthy eggs just fine. The problem was mechanical—because of blocked tubes, her husband's sperm never encountered her eggs. So in the fall of 1977, Steptoe checked her in to a hospital in Oldham and laparoscopically removed a naturally produced egg from her ovary, which he passed along to Edwards. Edwards fertilized Brown's egg in the laboratory using her husband's sperm, then returned it to her uterus two days later as a perfect, eight-celled embryo.

Nine months later, she gave birth to a healthy baby girl, giving hope to infertile couples around the world. Still, the unusual nature of her daughter's birth also left a legacy of suspicion and fear for her health and the health of her child.

Lesley Brown was not administered any pituitary-suppressive drugs or gonadotropin tainted with disease, and she had a healthy pregnancy and a routine cesarean birth. But even after her death, in 2012 (of complications after a gallbladder infection), she remains the object of curiosity and speculation. Google her, and one of the first suggestions is "Lesley Brown IVF cause of death."

On YouTube, if you search for "Follistim injection" or "Lupron injection," you'll get hundreds of results, most of them recorded by women in treatment for infertility. This is useful for new patients, like me, who have never self-administered shots, and some of the videos have thousands of views. The injections are given in kitchens and living rooms and dining rooms, in front of bathroom mirrors, sometimes by the women themselves and sometimes by their partners. Before starting IVF I watched dozens of these videos, not to learn to do my own injections but to feel a kind of kinship with these women as they tap their syringes free of air bubbles, swab their bellies, and hold the needle at just the right angle. In the backgrounds of the videos I watched were the messy signs of daily life you might find anywhere—piles of mail on the table, a television left on, houseplants growing toward a window—but there was a formality to their voices as they slowly narrated each step. *I have all of the stuff I need right here . . . See how I swab the top of the medicine bottle . . . Next I'll clean my skin . . . Ready, one, two, three.* Sometimes I could hear the commentary of an unseen partner, holding the camera: *Look at how brave, look at how tough.* I sensed that they were documenting something important—not the expense, not the pain, but the chance they were taking, the desire, the all-in commitment.

Richard injected me between six and seven every evening.

Preparing the injections—measuring and mixing the medication, drawing the solutions into the needle, tapping out the air
bubbles—took about twenty minutes, and during that time
our kitchen table was cluttered with papers, boxes, vials, and
syringes. He spread out the instructions from our clinic each
time, watched the online tutorial, checked and double-checked
the amounts before saying, "Okay, ready?" As with the well
drilling, there was an element of excess and surrender to this
experience that felt unfamiliar and frightening, but it was too
late to turn back.

I'd turn my head as soon as he swabbed my stomach with
alcohol, biting into a piece of dark chocolate—a trick I learned
from a friend, another woman who never imagined conception
this way. The shots didn't take long; I'd feel the needle pierce
my skin, then a stinging, and then it was over. Each one left
a pink mark that quickly faded, and sometimes a small, faint
bruise. Afterward I'd look for the injection sites under a strong
light, even though it was too early to know what was happening
beneath the skin.

It is not just the takeover of your body that makes IVF so
challenging, but the takeover of your schedule, your life. Every-
other-morning appointments, waiting by the phone for news
about the results of blood draws, timing injections precisely,
ordering more medication or procuring discounted or free left-
overs from women finished with their cycles: it all takes time.
While Richard came to every appointment and performed every
injection, I knew that if he had a sudden work emergency, he
would be able to step away. Infertility was our problem together,
but it was my body being treated, my body that had to attend
every appointment and accept the shots. I handed over my insurance card. I ordered the medicine and dealt with the pharmacy and changed my workout routine. I was dimly aware that
if I became pregnant, this imbalance would still exist, and would
become even more pronounced with a breast-fed newborn.

More than my body and my schedule, it took over my mind. I was always thinking of my possible pregnancy or looking out for superstitious tricks to bring it about. I watched the clock for 11:11, walked until I found good-luck clovers, prayed though I don't believe in God. I was always desirous and worried, never at peace. If it didn't work, we'd have more tries: six at most, three using fresh embryos and three with frozen embryos, if there were any left over from our other cycles. And if those didn't work—what then?

I tried not to think of what then.

Few studies have examined the effects of involuntary childlessness after medical treatment, but some psychologists have suggested that the myriad treatment options make it difficult for women to know when to stop. If Clomid doesn't work, maybe your ovaries will be more receptive to Femara. Or maybe you need an injectable gonadotropin and estrogen patches? If one IVF protocol fails, there are others, and if those fail too, you can try donor egg or surrogacy, provided you can pay the increasingly hefty bills. There is also the choice of clinics—a woman in Raleigh might interview doctors at four different practices; a New Yorker could see more than a dozen.

The availability of choices is known to decrease our happiness: gathering the information necessary to select among a range of options creates a sometimes paralyzing anxiety, and once we've chosen, we are prone to second-guessing and remorse. Reproductive medicine presents a twist to the choice paradox: while in treatment, patients report feeling hopeful, even excited, but each treatment cycle is just a few weeks long. Even the most advanced and expensive treatments offer a poor success rate: a thirty-five-year-old woman, on average, has a 31 percent chance of having a baby through a single IVF cycle. If unsuccessful, she must decide: try again? Try something new? The abundance of options also makes it more likely that she will blame herself, fearing that she has made the wrong choice or has taken too long to settle on the right one. Though I heard women in my support group state firmly that after the next cycle, they'd be done, studies of women who have completed unsuccessful courses of treatment suggest otherwise. The desire for a biological child does not fade into ambivalence or deepen into wise acceptance, post-treatment: it only grows stronger.

Despite worldwide attention and acclaim, it took Steptoe and Edwards two and a half years after Louise Brown's birth to open Bourn Hall, the world's second IVF clinic, in a renovated Jacobean mansion in Cambridge. Unlike Lesley Brown, Steptoe and Edwards knew all along that they were doing something remarkable, and they wanted an impressive home for the groundbreaking work they expected to continue.

Edwards, in particular, had great plans for his clinic: "IVF had to become large-scale, in a center providing the necessary clinical, scientific, consultative, nursing and counseling backup services, and even providing ward and dining facilities for the immense patient numbers on Steptoe's waiting list." He boasted that, though the clinic was not the first, it was the most beautiful. With its stately brick face, crenellated turrets, and engraved motto—JOUR DE MA VIE—Bourn Hall, still in operation today, looks more like an exclusive boarding school or university than it does a medical facility. John and Lesley Brown, who paid for their first appointment with Steptoe using winnings from a soccer pool, had been intimidated by the posh, fur-coat-wearing patients in the waiting room of his nondescript Oldham clinic. What would they have thought of Bourn Hall?

Our clinic, newly settled in to the third floor of a bland brick office building, looked more like a hotel for business travel, with furniture that appeared (but was not, in fact) comfortable, textured wallpaper patterned with ginkgo leaves and bamboo, soft recessed lighting. There was a Keurig coffeemaker stationed below a television tuned to CNN, and free tiny hand sanitizers in a basket. Plaques on the wall described the eco-friendly building practices—sustainable flooring, low-VOC paint. The receptionist's voice as she called each of us to the desk to sign paperwork and offer insurance cards (just in case) was low, discreet.

At the old clinic, we waited in chairs with mysterious stains, barely shielded from the rest of the hospital by leaf-dropping ficus trees. It was depressing and public but not unbearable. It felt as though we were there for a medical problem, which we were. The moneyed, leisurely atmosphere at the new place hardly reflected my own state of mind and didn't change it; I have never felt more vulnerable or hurried than I did in that waiting room. Though we were in a high-income suburb of Raleigh—increased proximity to a larger number of patients was another motivation behind the clinic's move—the other patients I saw looked like they might just as easily have been in the waiting room of a Patient First or in the terminal of an airport. No one was dressed to go back to a corporate job; everyone looked tired. I remember a man in a hockey jersey, a woman wearing an Aéropostale sweatshirt. We sat on the edges of our comfortable-looking chairs and listened for our names.

When I was a child, I had fantasies of sickness and treatment. Though I was rarely sick, my younger brother had severe asthma, and for a few years we were in and out of doctors' offices and hospitals. His resigned endurance of medication, shots, and breathing treatments looked valorous to me—he never cried and rarely complained, while I once required a sling after a vaccination. I can remember when they allergy-tested him, his skinny, pale back pricked and marked dozens of times, and how I coveted the marks (if not the pricks).

The nurses at my fertility clinic were gentle, but my veins were small, or they rolled to the side, or my blood pressure was too low. Kim, my favorite, humored me as I swung my arms to increase my heart rate, and still it took several tries to get a good stick. Kim was monitoring my estradiol, a measure of the estrogen secreted by my ovarian follicles. In an unmedicated cycle a woman might produce 200–300 pg/mL of estradiol from a single mature follicle. Thanks to my daily injections, I was superovulating, and we were waiting for my estradiol to rise above 2,000 before triggering ovulation. In the afternoons I waited for her phone call, when she'd tell me the result and whether I should adjust the dosage of my medication. Everything about my cycle was artificial and controlled, from the follicle-stimulating hormones that swelled my ovaries to the shot of human chorionic gonadotropin that would complete the maturation and time the release of my eggs so that the doctor could aspirate them into a hollow needle. Even the meeting of egg and sperm would be assisted by a doctor's steady hands—our embryologist would select "the fastest, strongest, best swimmers" and inject one into each mature oocyte.

In the exam room, I opened to a fresh page in my notebook and lay back on the table as the doctor stretched a condom over the transvaginal ultrasound transducer. A woman in my support group said she named this wand Simon, because you have to do what Simon says—but all I could think of was the recent fight in Virginia, my home state, over abortion. The pro-lifers wanted to require all women seeking abortions to have at least one transvaginal ultrasound before termination. Certainly this ultrasound was unnecessary, prohibitively expensive for many, and horribly invasive. Opponents also said it was painful, akin to state-sponsored rape. I lay on my back with my feet in stirrups; it was more uncomfortable to me to consider the distance between my circumstances and the circumstances of someone seeking an abortion than it was to receive this ultrasound. It barely hurt—I feel traitorous admitting that—but by then I must have had a dozen. I couldn't make myself picture what it would feel like to be internally prodded before terminating a pregnancy. I didn't try.

"You'll feel my touch," all of the nurses and some of the doctors would say before touching me. "Some pressure," they'd say, before turning the transducer's wand to the left or the right. Everything that touched me, as gentle and respectful as the nurses and doctors were, was nevertheless heavy with symbolic, perhaps inaccurate, meaning. The wand was a symbol of control and power; lying prone, feet in stirrups, I was the picture of submission. Watching the black-and-white images of an ultrasound machine, Richard and I were hopeful future parents. I wrote down the thickness of my endometrial lining (6 mm) and the approximate sizes of the six follicles on my right ovary (ranging from 11 to 12.5 mm), the four on my left (10 to 12.7 mm). The numbers meant little to me in real terms, but I knew from scanning message boards until my eyes burned that they were reassuring.

By the time Kim took my blood for a final estradiol level, a few days later, there was scar tissue on my veins. Even this was a metaphor, for the addiction I feared would take hold once we started down the path of assisted reproduction. One more cycle, one more treatment, until all our money and emotional resources were spent. Already I was addicted to Internet message boards, reading one on Momtastic.com's assisted-conception page each morning about the current IVF cycles of women from all over the world, Linesmanswife and Worriedone and Everhopeful and Mamali. "Praying we are going to be 3rd time lucky," wrote africaqueen, the thirty-one-year-old woman from Liverpool who started the conversation. She and her Nigerian-born husband had already exhausted England's public funding for IVF with two failed cycles and were counting on a loan from family—her father's life savings, she said—to pay for their final round. She had more than six thousand posts to

Momtastic forums and was tirelessly upbeat and encouraging, despite her past disappointments. "Who else is gearing up for the patter of tiny feet? This thread is gonna be full of PMAs and also BFPs!" I had to look up PMA; it stands for "positive mental attitude," a difficult state of mind to maintain, given the ups and downs of the average ART cycle, when almost every day brings news about estradiol levels (too high? too low?), the numbers and sizes of follicles, the thickness of the uterine lining. This news, bad or good, is so specialized that it takes another person who has been through IVF to understand. "Lucky threads" like the one africaqueen created allow women to feel, at their most vulnerable and isolated, a sense of community that they probably could not with their girlfriends, mothers, or sisters. On their lunch breaks or in a spare moment, they can commiserate and seek advice and cheer each other on. They send each other sticky vibes and hopes for big, healthy follies and strong, beautiful embies. Their posts are embellished with animated emoticons—smiley faces offering hugs, smiley faces dancing or crying, pregnancy tests with two flashing pink lines. I was a lurker—I never posted, had no handle or icon to identify myself with—but I sent them lucky vibes as well as I could.

On the morning of our last scheduled ultrasound, my estradiol was 2,248 pg/mL, and a doctor I'd seen only once or twice, known in our support group for her brisk bedside manner, counted ten large follicles. This would be a win for most of the women on the message board, but I worried it wouldn't be enough. The doctor said things looked "good" but didn't elaborate. We were given precise written instructions about how to measure out the hCG injection that will mature my eggs so they can be retrieved. "Pay attention," she said, tapping the page as if we might be daydreaming.

Two mornings later, the day of our retrieval, it was raining and cold. We arrived at 7:45 a.m. with a plate of cookies for the staff and were led to a part of the clinic we'd never seen before, which looked reassuringly medical—more like the presurgical area of a hospital than a hotel. They gave me a gown to change into, and a nurse named Lenora attached my IV. It took her three tries to find a vein; I turned my head while she searched, and didn't complain.

A few minutes later I was clutching my gown closed behind me, wheeling my IV to the retrieval room. It was very much like the image I feared for years—a long hallway, all the doors closed, with IVF at the end. But I was far from alone, and it didn't feel routine or workaday or cold. Kim helped me onto the table. Dr. Young was there, and Dr. Ramos, the effusive Brazilian embryologist I interviewed when we first seriously considered IVF, greeted me with a jaunty wave that morning. Richard waited just one room away; he'd be there to help me back into my clothes and drive me home. I lay down, counted backward, and fell asleep.

Michelle, our embryologist, called with news the next morning— of the thirteen eggs they retrieved, eleven were mature and ten fertilized. She told me they wouldn't check the embryos again until day three, when I could choose to transfer or to wait until day five. I recorded this in my notebook, then went for a walk by the river and found four four-leaf clovers. I saw a bald eagle perched in the huge pine tree across from our neighborhood easement, near her nest. I recorded these things too, and pressed a single clover into the notebook.

On Momtastic's lucky thread, Mells54 was PUPO (pregnant until proven otherwise), a term of optimism many women use after transfer. Ashknowsbest produced twenty-five mature eggs; indeedaseed, now pregnant, only had three. The general consensus: it only takes one. Will eating the core of a pineapple help with implantation? Will eating too much cause contractions? LPEAR, now pregnant, recommended Brazil nuts. Africaqueen, still struggling to finance her cycle, uncharacteristically reported

feeling "very down" and taking a trip with her father to the zoo
to see baby elephants, a baby meerkat, and a baby anteater.
Sunshine24 wrote: "Work was soooo crazy and stressful today
though and they are making cuts left and right and I may end
up losing my job in a few months but I cant even focus or think
about that right now, not the most important thing I have going
on, by far!" Africaqueen had an idea from her last cycle: what if
she organized a "secret sister chain," like a secret Santa through
the mail? "It is a lovely little game to cheer the spirit and you
dont need to send anything expensive, it can be anything that
will raise a smile," she wrote. "We used to send a baby item,
cards, sweets, keepsakes, anything at all to help cheer us up on
this journey."

Lesley Brown entered into her treatment unaware of its
remarkable nature, unable to research the procedure, consult
with other women in support groups, or join any secret sister-
hoods. Though she envisioned hundreds of other women se-
cretly giving birth to babies who'd been implanted by Steptoe,
infertility, in her imagination, made her abnormal. *How long
have you been married?* newcomers to the cheese factory where
she worked would ask. The next question was always the same:
How many children? Brown had even given up the chance for
better-paying work to avoid having to explain her blocked fallopian tubes all over again.

And so it was a revelation for Brown to share a hospital room
with another of Steptoe's patients while they waited for retrieval, transfer, and a pregnancy test: "Having imagined for so
long that I was the only one in existence who couldn't have a
baby, it had been amazing to meet someone in the same position as me," she wrote. The two women talked about how childlessness isolated them and planned visits once they each got
their babies. "Being the same age," Brown said, "our children
were bound to be friends."

When her roommate got her period before she could take the pregnancy test, Brown was left alone again. Steptoe's patients had been segregated from the rest of the hospital's maternity ward, but she didn't feel like talking to the other women— some of whom were busy giving birth, yelling and moaning— anyway. John brought her a portable television, which she barely watched. "I couldn't concentrate on anything except what was happening inside me," she said.

So she took her meals alone, visited daily with Dr. Steptoe, and prayed.

Richard and I had a phone conference with Dr. Young two days after the retrieval. The standard number of embryos transferred by someone my age was two, but I was eligible, Dr. Young mentioned, to transfer three. We told him about our desire to transfer a single embryo, a choice made then, at our clinic, by only 3 percent of patients in my age bracket. We wanted to avoid the risk of twins—not so much of twin car seats and double strollers and double college tuition bills, but the risk to my body, the risk to the fetuses carried within.

Waiting until day five would make it clearer which of the embryos was most "competent," or likely to develop normally. Not every embryo makes it to day five—some divide perfectly, into round morulas on day four and complex blastulas on day five—but others short-circuit somehow, dividing unevenly or stopping division entirely. Waiting would allow us to choose the best one, I insisted to Dr. Young, who countered that my uterus—part of the reproductive system he spent weeks taking over—was actually the best place for the embryos, which was why most women my age chose to transfer two embryos on day three. *Their natural environment,* I think he said. Richard scribbled notes in red pen on plain white paper, but he didn't write this part down.

Dr. Young had a formula: if three times as many embryos as we wished to transfer (for us, that meant three competent embryos) were developing normally on day three, we could wait.

Here is what I wrote down when Michelle called on day three:

> *10 embryos*
> *7 8-cell*
> *1 9-cell*
> *1 11-cell*
> *1 5-cell*
> *4 look perfect*
> *4 look almost perfect*
> *1 has 1 slightly bigger cell but is appropriately celled*
> *1 is 5-cell (may make it to blast on day 6)*

I wondered which one they would transfer. I wished I could see photographs. I wished they could do all their development inside the laboratory, which I had come to trust more than my body.

"There's something really wrong about the fact that my body doesn't function in the way that it was born to function," confided a woman in Marni Rosner's study of involuntarily childless women. "There is a sense . . . that my body failed me and I try not to sort of allow that to take over my mindset because it's not particularly healthy, but I do feel that . . . in certain circles, makes me feel like I don't have any credibility."

ART patients often see their bodies as suspect and view medication and surgery as the body's replacement rather than its assistant. Doctors who glibly tell us they can get us pregnant, or that they will take over our cycles, feed this system of belief. Lesley Brown, who spurned her husband's sexual advances for years after her diagnosis of infertility, telling him to find a "normal" woman, blamed her ovaries while she waited for Dr. Steptoe to retrieve her egg. The other two women in her ward had already had their operations, and she worried that her chance had passed. "But, as it turned out, it was just my body's fault," she wrote. "I was later in reaching a state of ovulation than the other girls."

Our bodies are miracles is a message most often given to two groups of people: children entering puberty and women preparing for childbirth. It makes sense to lie to children facing years of bodily inconvenience (monthly bleeding, wet dreams, unexpected erections) or to women facing many hours of agony, but evolutionary biology suggests that our bodies are not really the miracles we proclaim them to be but jury-rigged compromises. Like the physiology of all living things, human physiology has evolved to be not perfect but only good enough to allow individuals to survive and pass along our genes. "Neither we nor any other species have ever been a seamless match with the environment," writes evolutionary biologist Marlene Zuk in *Paleofantasy,* her book about the ways we romanticize nature and evolution. "Instead, our adaptation is more like a broken zipper, with some teeth that align and others that gape apart." Our fishlike vertebrate plan makes us prone to hiccups and hernias; unassisted childbirth has a high mortality rate, thanks to the large brains of our babies. We waste all kinds of things that take energy to produce, like our monthly allotment of eggs or sperm, and live (we hope) beyond our reproductive capacity. We each carry inside of us a relatively useless organ—the appendix— which at any moment could rupture and threaten our lives.

Before the advent of reproductive medicine, an infertile woman could not expect to pass along her genes—her body was not only not perfect, but not even good enough by the metrics of evolution. Edwards and Steptoe were frequently criticized because their work did not cure infertility—their patients were just as infertile after IVF, whether or not they gave birth. Edwards, who would receive the Nobel Prize in medicine

in 2010, handily brushed off the complaints: what about spec-
tacles, false teeth, and heart transplants?

We blame our bodies because we idealize them; we apply
a metaphor—*miracle*—that does not fit. The first IVF baby,
Louise Brown, was called a miracle too—as well as a freak of
nature, a test-tube baby, and the first step onto a slippery ethical
slope. Well-wishers from around the world sent Louise cards
and gifts, but her Bristol neighbors would often peer curiously
into her pram, her mother said, as if they expected her to be
made of glass.

Our Miracle Called Louise: A Parents' Story is the full title
of Lesley and John Brown's memoir. They each have their say,
alternating chapters in a candid and conversational style, and
spend most of the book describing their loving but rocky relationship, which began when John noticed sixteen-year-old
Lesley at a café in Bristol and said, admiringly, "What a cracker."
Reading it, I felt a little impatient to get to the IVF treatment—
the miracle part—and then let down by the lack of detail there,
compared with the bustling chapters about hanging out in cafés
and sleeping in railcars. But for them, this was the story of how
they came to be Louise's parents—a story that begins not in a
clinic's waiting room but with the extraordinary series of random events that leads any of us to our partner.

"Louise is special because she would never have been born
at all in the normal way," Lesley writes near the end. "It was a
miracle that I was chosen to have her."

I imagine, if given the choice between the birth they had and
a more conventional one, that John and Lesley Brown would have
gladly repeated all the turmoil they experienced on the path to
their daughter: the waiting, the financial hardship, the tabloid
attention, all culminated in the one and only Louise. After the
surrogate birth of his IVF-conceived son, Andrew Solomon felt
an even deeper connection to the hundreds of parents he interviewed for *Far from the Tree* and reflected that parenting makes

the subjective, which emphasizes fate over randomness, more real than objective truths. Our children, according to Solomon, "are the children we had to have; we could have had no others. They will never seem to us to be happenstance; we love them because they are our destiny."

"All that really matters is that we've got her," wrote John Brown thirty-five years earlier, with less eloquence but the same conviction. "I couldn't be without Louise now."

On the day of transfer, Dr. Young brought us a photograph of the blastocyst they chose, "the prettiest one," the embryologist reported, that she had seen all year. This handing over of image (or images, for women transferring two or more embryos) is part of the ritual of ART; if you get this far, it is the proof of what the takeover accomplished, the closest thing to those fetal ultrasounds posted to fridges and Facebook pages. I wasn't sure how I would feel looking at a mass of cells in medium—let down? ambivalent? *motherly?* But I clung to the embryologist's words; I wrote them down in my notebook before I even looked at the photograph.

I'd seen enough of these images online, in medical journals, and in Dr. Ramos's office to know that this was a good-looking embryo. The grainy black-and-white picture showed a mostly hollow sphere with many cells in the center, an already complex planet floating in space. Each cell of the inner mass, at this point, could become almost anything: heart, brain, lung. The embryo was hatching, just starting to break free of the smooth walls of the zona pellucida in preparation for implantation. At the bottom of the image, the embryologist had written my last name and the date.

Some clinics routinely offer sedation during embryo transfer, usually a Valium, and they'll let you play soft music if you like. The theory is that it relaxes you, so your body is better prepared to receive your embryo. This sounds like a thoughtful, considerate touch, like the little coffee-and-tea station in the lobby, but in reality it's often necessary. Some women who make it this far are on their third, fourth, or sixth IVF. Sometimes they are transferring embryos with little chance of implantation. Some of them have had miscarriages and D & Cs and traumatic ectopic pregnancies, and the padded stirrups and instruments they use in this room are full of meaning that has to be blocked out if they are to go forward.

Richard and I were lucky to have had none of those memories or bad experiences, just our years of waiting, and the takeover had gone better than we expected. Entering the transfer room, which days before had been my retrieval room, I didn't need a pill or music. This first time, which I hoped was my only time, I didn't want anything buffering the experience.

It was quiet enough to hear the humming of machines, and there was a strange formality as Dr. Young read my name aloud—an oddly low-tech precaution, given our circumstances. I held as still as I could while he threaded a thin catheter past my cervix. Kim, standing next to me, pressed an ultrasound wand into my stomach so he could select just the right spot. There was a spark of light on the monitor.

"There it is!" said Dr. Young. "Your embryo."

Richard and I squeezed hands. Nothing about this experience had been what we expected when we thought of having children, or even when we first guessed that the road to parenthood might be a long one. It was more uncomfortable and expensive than we imagined, and less private—there were three other people in the room with us, plus family and friends who would want to know, in less than two weeks, if our IVF was successful.

Then the doctor, the nurse, and the embryologist all left, and it was just us: two people who might never have met, had these struggles, and made this embryo. A clock ticked on the wall, but we knew that no one would rush us. Though we were usually talkative with each other, even in examination rooms with my feet in stirrups, a shyness and reserve came over us as we considered the seriousness of what we'd done. We might have a baby in nine months, or more choices to make. For now we waited, again.

Birth Stories

•••

Todd Jensen proposed to Gabe Faibish on a warm evening in May 2012. They were at Lantern, a romantic pan-Asian restaurant in Chapel Hill, the sort of place where every pea shoot and pork chop has a local pedigree and the light is low and flattering. They'd walked to dinner from their recently remodeled house, and, though the night was an auspicious one—the ninth anniversary of their first date—Gabe was not expecting a proposal of marriage. "I thought we were just trying to make it through the week," Gabe remembered, a little ruefully. "It was one of our 'passionate periods.'" Gabe, a writer and actor used to long considerations of character and motivation, said *Yes, but not now.* Todd, a self-assured public-health researcher and professor, heard *No.* They walked home in a deflated, wistful mood, walked their Labrador, and went to bed.

For Gabe, the desirability of marriage, and the idea that he might live happily inside that institution, was relatively new. He didn't come out until his early thirties, in graduate school, and before that had spent years in a committed and loving relationship with a woman, struggling all the while with his sexuality. For a long time—even after he met Todd, on a picnic with friends in Central Park—he thought that being gay meant certain kinds of family structures were closed to him. He would not get married, would not have a house with a dog and a yard and children.

Gabe deliberated, mostly internally, for the next several months, and finally decided: he was ready. They married the next June, in Brooklyn—same-sex marriage was constitutionally forbidden in North Carolina—in the garden of a favorite Carroll Gardens restaurant. The ceremony was Jewish with Buddhist touches: their guests chanted the Buddhist Prayer of Loving Kindness after Gabe and Todd stomped the glass that symbolized the start of their new life together, and their *chuppah* was made of both Gabe's grandfather's *tallith* and a Buddhist prayer shawl Todd uses during meditation. Months later, they started talking about kids, an even bigger, more important question for both of them than matrimony.

They discussed the question for more than a year. Gabe wondered what their new life would look like, what child-care responsibilities would mean for his day job and his writing life, how parenting would affect their relationship. After a hard, soul-searching winter—during which he read a lot, joined a swim clinic, talked intensively with close friends about his doubts and desires about becoming a parent—Gabe decided affirmatively. He wanted to raise a child, an undertaking he could imagine only with Todd at his side.

"The history of marriage is one of both continuity and change," wrote Supreme Court justice Anthony Kennedy two years after Gabe and Todd tied the knot, in the majority opinion of *Obergefell v. Hodges,* the historic decision that legalized same-sex marriage nationwide. Kennedy's opinion, joined by Justices Ruth Bader Ginsburg, Elena Kagan, Stephen Breyer, and Sonia Sotomayor, referred to changes such as the abandonment of coverture and the decline of arranged marriage, but also the growing reality and public recognition of different kinds of family structures, including same-sex couples who cannot or do not have children, as well as couples who adopt or parent biological children. "Changed understandings of marriage are characteristic of a

Nation where new dimensions of freedom become apparent to new generations," wrote Kennedy.

In advance of the decision, many SCOTUS watchers predicted that the court's reasoning would rest both on a non-procreative view of marriage, established in an earlier case about contraceptive access, as well as on this expanded definition of family. The split feels like a natural one to me—it makes sense that access to something as varied and complicated as marriage would have all kinds of reasoning behind it. But some legal scholars saw the potential for other avenues of legal restriction, as well as a natural alliance between same-sex and some opposite-sex couples who seek ART to build their families.

"As same-sex couples have gained access to marriage, some who opposed same-sex marriage have shifted their views, expressing support for marriage equality while attempting to limit its impact," wrote Douglas NeJaime, a professor of law at UCLA, in an essay written in advance of the *Obergefell* decision for the *Yale Law Journal*. "In particular, some now accept same-sex marriage while maintaining their commitment to biological, gender-differentiated parenting. In other words, they abandon their opposition to same-sex couples' exclusion from marriage without abandoning a chief argument used to support that exclusion."

NeJaime warned that, even as marriage equality becomes the law of the land, "new sites of conflict are emerging." He cited David Blankenhorn, a prominent social conservative and founder of the Institute for American Values, who changed his mind about same-sex marriage—he testified in support of California's Proposition 8, the 2008 constitutional amendment prohibiting same-sex marriage, but later came out in support of federal recognition—while continuing to maintain that "no same-sex couple, married or not, can ever under any circumstances combine biological, social and legal parenthood into one bond." Parenthood by same-sex couples would always be lesser, Blankenhorn insisted, because of biology. His organization funded and published a study of young adults conceived through sperm donation called "My Daddy's Name Is Donor" and works to restrict ART based on the belief that donor-conceived children fare less well than others and have rights that are not being protected.

NeJaime calls family formation "the next frontier" of sexual-orientation equality. On a personal level, that's true for Gabe and Todd, who face a number of restrictions and opportunities, both biological and legal, as they consider how to have a child.

Gabe and I are members of the same four-person writing group; we meet once a month at a small, treehouse-like café on the outskirts of Chapel Hill and often start with gossip and personal news. I remember when Gabe first told us that he and Todd were considering parenthood; he confessed his ambivalence, and another member of our group warned him about needing to be really sure before taking the leap. She's a gracious and thoughtful woman who had children relatively young—her kids are now at that age where they seem at once scarily independent and also impossibly time consuming—and she must have thought, *Uh-oh, do you really know what you're getting into?*

But I related, through my own years of indecision, and sent Gabe what I hoped was an encouraging email the next morning. By then I'd had my daughter and was something of an evangelist for parenthood. But also, I hope, for ambivalence and the way a complicated understanding of the future allows you to live for a while with both possibilities: have a baby and stagger through a year or two of distraction and sleeplessness and joy, or continue a child-free life of freedom and romance. Adopting or making use of reproductive technologies—the only way Gabe and Todd would become parents—means a long period of careful planning, of waiting. I don't know anyone who has embarked upon

either adoption or ART without some degree of ambivalence
and second-guessing.

"Family happens incrementally," writes legal scholar Martha
Ertman in *Love's Promises,* a book that exalts the power of contracts in family planning, especially for what she calls "Plan B"
families, which are created in uncommon ways—through ART,
adoption, family blending, or same-sex or single parenting. By
Plan B, Ertman says, she does not mean that these kinds of
families represent a second or lesser choice; she means instead
to replace "disdain or condescension with a . . . morally neutral
claim that society and people individually are better off when
we can choose when, how, and with whom to have a family."
Ertman's own family was created through donor insemination
and contractual parenting—her son's genetic father is also a
close friend and coparent. After Walter's birth, Ertman and
Victor, the child's father, each married same-sex partners, and
Walter now has two stepparents in his life. In *Love's Promises,*
the incremental creation of family refers both to the way Walter
has accrued his parents and also to the transforming nature of
parenthood: "Walter's birth made me a biological mother," she
writes, "but only changing, feeding, loving, and worrying about
him made me a mom."

In a larger way, the choices available to LGBT families have
happened incrementally too. Just a generation ago, many gay
men felt as Gabe once did about "traditional" family life—it
was unavailable to them, not only biologically but also socially.
Same-sex marriage, advances in reproductive technology, and
more liberal adoption laws have opened doors to some people
that were once sealed shut, and the people walking through
them now are often amazed at the rapid evolution that has happened in their lifetimes. In the concluding chapter of *Far From
the Tree,* Andrew Solomon writes, "For a long time, children
used to make me sad. The origin of my sadness was somewhat

obscure to me, but I think it came most from how the absence of children in the lives of gay people had repeatedly been held up to me as my tragedy. Children were the most important thing in the world, and so they were mascots for my failure."

I also grew up indoctrinated into a belief system that put children at life's center, and when I thought I wouldn't have children, I wanted a vastly different life, one that wouldn't remind me constantly of what I didn't have. Other people's children made me sad, too—not the children themselves but the way the parents held them up (rightfully but also, to my eyes, smugly) as the core of their existence.

Now I have a daughter, and Solomon has four children—two are his husband's genetic kids, conceived with lesbian friends; one is a child he fathered and coparents with a close female friend (similar to the arrangement Ertman describes with Victor), and his youngest is his genetic son, born to a surrogate who is also one of the mothers of his husband's genetic children. All of the children I've mentioned here—my daughter, Ertman's son, Solomon and his husband's daughters and sons—were born through some form of ART, without which we would not have been able to form our Plan B families. Ertman describes the gleeful sense of "getting away with something" she felt at the fertility clinic with Victor, "so different from the embarrassment and inadequacy" she imagined in the minds of the straight couples around them. "For gay people," she writes, "simply being here is a triumph."

It took me longer to feel this way, but now I am empowered by ART, too—not only by its outcome, the wonder of life with my daughter and ability to choose when or if I might have another child, but more abstractly by the way ART requires a decision, a commitment, the way it foils the limited human body. The way it draws me into common cause with people like Solomon and Ertman.

. . .

How to begin? Gabe and Todd wondered as they made the decision to become parents. For LGBT couples, the question has long been more complicated than for straight couples pursuing Plan B families. Post-*Obergefell,* adoption became more accessible in all states except Mississippi, which forbade same-sex adoption until a federal court ruling lifted the unconstitutional ban. But several states have introduced bills allowing agencies providing foster-care and adoption services to discriminate on religious grounds, and only seven states explicitly protect LGBT families from discrimination by foster-care agencies. Before the 2015 Supreme Court decision, some states would not allow such an adoption at all, and families were forced into compromises that did not protect parents or kids in the case of medical emergencies, educational decisions, inheritance, and other matters straight adoptive parents take for granted.

In North Carolina, as in other states, same-sex marriage and LGBT parenting rights have been intricately linked, even as same-sex couples parented long before they could access the same rights and recognitions as straight parents. As an amicus brief filed in support of *Obergefell* argued, same-sex couples are three times more likely to parent adopted or foster children.

Shawn Long, director of operations at Equality NC, a nonprofit organization dedicated to LGBT rights, became a father eight years ago, when he and his partner adopted a five-year-old boy from the foster-care system. "His name is *Isaiah,*" Shawn told me, with the same slight pause and proud emphasis I use when pronouncing my daughter's name. "He's my heart."

Shawn and his partner, Craig Johnson, were the first gay men to seek adoption through foster care in Wake County, North Carolina, and, while they found that the social-services professionals and other couples in their foster-adoption education program were welcoming and supportive, Shawn and Craig were also the last couple in their cohort to be matched by social workers with a child. As an unmarried couple—same-sex marriage was still unrecognized in North Carolina—they were unable to adopt their son together, even though they'd been a foster family by then for six months. They decided together that Craig would be the adoptive parent, and, although they established protective legal paperwork and continued to live as before, it pained Shawn to go "from a foster parent to a total legal stranger," he said. Shawn and Craig joined several other plaintiffs in a lawsuit filed by the ACLU challenging North Carolina's constitutional amendment forbidding same-sex marriage.

And they won. On October 10, 2014, a federal judge ruled North Carolina's same-sex marriage ban unconstitutional. Shawn and Craig had planned to be among the first couples in line at the magistrate's office, but, as it happened, family life intervened—Isaiah had an out-of-town soccer tournament that day. They were married the following Monday, with Isaiah in attendance, and now have the same rights as any other soccer dads. "We've been together twenty years," Shawn said, "but we're looking forward to our first anniversary."

As in *Obergefell v. Hodges,* the presence of children in the lives of the North Carolina plaintiffs was a significant factor in the way the case appeared to the public. Amendment 1, the state's primary-season ballot initiative banning same-sex marriage, passed overwhelmingly in 2012, but since then LGBT families, with their underlying Plan B structures, have become more outspoken and visible. "Discrimination is an education issue," Shawn told me. "When you can say, 'These are our families. We are parents. These are our children. We're trying to protect them,' people's hearts are more open."

Still, he noted, same-sex couples often face discrimination and prejudice when they seek adoptions—from social workers who might think a heterosexual couple would make better parents, or private agencies that willfully discriminate. This potentially treacherous landscape gave Gabe and Todd pause. Some of the largest American domestic adoption agencies refuse to work with LGBT couples and individuals (the largest, Bethany Christian Services, pledges to make decisions "consistent with Biblical principles" and does not work with LGBT couples); following *Obergefell,* it's possible additional states will pass so-called religious-liberty laws allowing adoption agencies to refuse placement of children with same-sex couples (Michigan passed such a law in June, before the Supreme Court decision). And, according to a Human Rights Campaign overview of LGBT adoption choices, thanks to cultural prejudices and discriminatory international laws, "it is very difficult to pursue an international adoption as an openly same-sex couple, or as an openly single LGBT person." Many of the most popular countries for adoptive parents from the United States (Guatemala, China, Ethiopia, South Korea, and Russia) explicitly prohibit same-sex couples and single parents from adopting; neither of the two countries Richard and I considered (Ethiopia and Haiti) would have allowed Gabe and Todd to adopt.

For Gabe and Todd to have a genetically related child would require surrogacy, an approach to conception so expensive and legally complex that it has become the primary focus of more than one boutique law firm. A major source of this legal complexity is the variance of laws from state to state, and in North Carolina, the law is particularly unclear: no statute regulates gestational surrogacy, in which an embryo is created with a donor egg and gestated by a contractually bound surrogate.

For Gabe, having a genetically linked child is emotionally compelling. His father, an only child, is a Holocaust survivor; Gabe's mother is an only child too. But, more than a desire to continue the family line, Gabe said, what he and Todd really want is "to raise a human being from moment one." The best way to achieve this goal, they decided, is gestational surrogacy. They agreed that Gabe would provide the male gametes—a genetic relationship was less important to Todd—and he began

the screening process, getting tested for heritable genetic ab-
normalities at a local clinic. The pornography selection in the
clinic's sperm-sample room was "comically heteronormative,"
Gabe said, and the instructions about washing up were confusing, but everything worked out—he had strong swimmers and
is not a genetic carrier for any of the diseases more common in
Jewish bloodlines.

How and where to find a surrogate was the big question.
Their close female friends were mostly too old or encumbered
to ask or offer, and they didn't have good candidates in their families either. They knew other couples who had hired American
surrogates, but this had involved contracting with agencies and
surrogates in other states and was also staggeringly expensive:
about $150,000 in legal, agency, medical, and surrogate fees.

Gabe's family is Israeli American, and he has a friend in
Israel, Doron Mamet, who founded an international surrogacy
operation, Tammuz, that matches intended parents, mostly
from Israel but also the United States, many of them gay men,
with surrogates in the United States, India, and at that time in
Nepal. Gabe and Todd were interested in the Nepal program,
in which Indian women (India prohibits surrogacy on behalf
of same-sex couples) travel alone or with their families to live
in Nepal under a medical tourist visa (Nepal prohibits surrogacy by its own citizens but not, at the time, by foreigners). The
women are impregnated with embryos created from egg donors
from South Africa (egg donation is illegal in Israel) and live in
apartments in Kathmandu during the pregnancy, where they
receive the same prenatal care as Western mothers. The practical and emotional challenges inherent in this program—the
need for expensive and time-consuming travel, waiting while
one's child is gestated in a poor country halfway around the
world—are reflected in its cost, about half the fees associated with American gestational surrogacy. Tammuz caters to
gay men in particular and was founded in response to Israel's

restrictive surrogacy laws—only heterosexual couples are allowed to contract with Israeli surrogates.

"I wanted to be a parent my whole life," Mamet tells a hopeful couple over Skype in a scene from *Google Baby,* a 2010 documentary about international surrogacy. "There is no reason because of what someone might think, that I am not worthy of being a parent, for me not to be a parent. So I went and became a parent. And I would be happy to help others to become parents."

It's hard to watch *Google Baby* without some degree of unease, and reviews were critical of the international baby market it exposes. Still, Mamet mentions the film (a 2011 Emmy award winner) on Tammuz International's home page, as if the attention it generated were a sign of his company's quality or, perhaps, as a way of owning up to the controversial nature of his work. I spoke to him over Skype, and he told me that, while *Google Baby* looks like one narrative, the film tells in fact three unconnected stories—the story of his meetings with clients, the story of American egg donors not connected to Tammuz, and the story of Indian surrogates who have never worked with Tammuz.

Critics responding to the film—and to international surrogacy in general—take issue with the lack of regulation surrounding the process, the Indian surrogate mothers' lack of economic and medical agency (payments are made to their husbands, and they are routinely given medically unnecessary cesarean sections), the blithely businesslike attitude of an IVF clinician/obstetrician who appears in the film (she takes a phone call while stitching up a postbirth surrogate), and the way the whole process reads like a metaphor for globalization at its most extreme.

Though recorded forms of surrogacy date back to the Old Testament, when Sarah instructed Abraham to have a child with their maidservant, contemporary views of contractual surrogacy tend to emphasize its dystopian and futuristic qualities, as well as people's discomfort with any agreement that would compel a gestational or genetic mother to give away her baby. I remember reading Margaret Atwood's *The Handmaid's Tale* when I was in seventh grade (I borrowed the novel from my mother, possibly without her knowledge) and feeling terrified by the society she envisions: a militaristic Christian theocracy in which wealthy and powerful couples force fertile young women to live in their homes, have sex with the husbands, and bear children for the couples to raise as their own.

Atwood has written that she felt a great deal of anxiety before the book was released, but it was critically well received and quickly became a bestseller. It was published in the United States in February 1986, coincidentally just one month before the birth of "Baby M," the child at the center of a court battle that brought ethical and legal considerations of surrogacy to worldwide attention. Baby M was born to Mary Beth Whitehead, a Jersey Shore woman who entered into a traditional (as opposed to gestational) surrogacy agreement with William and Elizabeth Stern, an infertile couple from prosperous Tenafly. Whitehead was inseminated with William Stern's sperm and decided at the birth that she wanted to dissolve their $10,000 agreement and keep the child. The case—which ultimately returned Baby M to the Sterns while preserving visitation rights for Whitehead—was for many a reminder of what can happen when poor women are bodily exploited, as in Atwood's novel, by the wealthy. In response, several U.S. states banned compensated surrogacy entirely. Gestational surrogacy, in which the surrogate carries no genetic link to the child, became the default practice in places like California, where compensated surrogacy was still legal.

Many feminists responding to the Baby M case sided with Ms. Whitehead, who was subject, via the custody case, to a troubling assessment of her fitness as a mother that evaluated everything from the toys she gave her baby to her own choice to dye her hair. A group of women writers from New York drafted an open letter that declared, "By these standards we are all unfit mothers." It was signed by more than one hundred women, including Betty Friedan, Gloria Steinem, Nora Ephron, and Meryl Streep.

I would have sided with Mary Beth Whitehead too. I still would—it's hard to imagine that she could have predicted how she'd feel giving up her child when she signed away her rights before the child was even conceived, before she carried it in her body for nine long months. That doesn't mean I don't also feel empathy for the intended parents—especially Elizabeth Stern, a pediatrician whose legal status as a mother was revoked and unacknowledged by the courts, even as she raised the child to adulthood in her home—and for Baby M, whose first months of life were full of globally documented public upheaval.

Martha Ertman insists it is possible to arrange surrogacy-for-hire that protects the surrogate, the intended parents, and the child: make sure it's gestational and in a state that honors surrogacy contracts, and you won't have a problem, because "people generally give and get what they expect." But when your baby is gestated thousands of miles away, by an uneducated woman in a developing country, how do you know that your surrogate is fully informed, that she isn't subject to exploitation? How do you know that she won't feel an abiding sorrow when the infant is carried out of the delivery room?

Gabe told me what he hoped, and what he'd been told by Mamet—that the women in Nepal lived comfortably, that they were able to make their lives better, to buy houses and educate their own children. But, he admitted, "you don't know. You can't know."

Mamet, whose two children were birthed by American surrogates, told me that his only ethical concern about using Indian women as Tammuz surrogates is one of choice—he isn't sure that the women aren't pressured by their husbands and families to do the work. "I can't tell," he said. "But I can't tell that about an American [woman] either."

Tammuz International made the news again in April 2015, when a magnitude 7.8 earthquake shook Nepal, killing 8,800 people and injuring more than 23,000. None of the company's Kathmandu-based surrogates or staff were injured, but a number of babies were born during the quake's aftermath, which included, for a time, powerful aftershocks every fifteen to twenty minutes. A few babies were born prematurely, and all survived, thanks to dedicated Nepali nurses who kept them warm and safe in heated cars in the hospital's parking lot. Some babies had been born days and weeks before and were living already with their intended parents, mostly Israeli couples, who were still in the process of obtaining the passports and birth certificates they needed to take their babies home.

Nepal is a popular tourist destination for Israelis, who are attracted to the beautiful scenery and the chance to hike Mt. Everest. Because of Israel's restrictive antigay surrogacy laws, and the growing business Doron Mamet founded, it also became the go-to destination for a practically and ethically complicated form of medical tourism. All told, there were 229 Israeli hikers, tourists, parents, and newborns in and around the earthquake's epicenter. Israel's government dispatched rescue teams and set up field camps to take care of quake victims. It evacuated the Israeli citizens, including the vulnerable newborns, but left the Indian surrogates—at least fifteen postbirth and more than eighty who were still pregnant.

How to read this story? For some, Israel's airlift of only its own citizens was an example of Western callousness and chauvinism, the field hospitals simply a cover for an exploitative baby market. For others—especially the parents of the newborns—it was a chance to expose the discrimination that allows only heterosexual couples to build families through surrogacy at home. But the story was also reported widely because it just sounds so exotic and strange—sperm from Israel, eggs from South Africa, surrogates from India, an earthquake in Nepal. On NPR's website, a photo of two hospital-gowned fathers holding their tiny son appeared with the caption "Now this is an international baby."

When he heard about the earthquake, Gabe asked Todd if he would still go through with the surrogacy in Nepal, provided things went back to normal. Todd said yes, and Gabe agreed. But going back to normal would mean more than rebuilding hospitals or getting past aftershocks (a strong one hit Nepal just two weeks later, killing another two hundred people). For the program to continue, it would have to survive the increased scrutiny that the earthquake and baby airlift generated. Thailand, another low-regulation developing country that once had a thriving surrogacy market, banned international surrogacy in 2015 after two major scandals: the alleged abandonment of a child with Down syndrome by an Australian couple (his surrogate mother is now raising him), and the bizarre case of a Japanese man who fathered sixteen children through Thai surrogates.

Continuing international surrogacy in Nepal would depend on how the story was read: Did Nepal need better fertility-tourism regulations? Should it be in the business of surrogacy at all? Does Israel need to change its own laws so that everyone can access surrogacy?

These questions remind me of our experience considering international adoption. The programs we could afford with the shortest wait times and youngest children were also the least regulated. Did I think those countries should suspend or slow their programs? Yes, I did. Was I disappointed when I heard that they had? Yes, I was.

Most forms of Plan B family making include contracts of one kind or another. At the beginning of our IVF cycle, Richard and I signed contracts with an agency that wrote our cost-share agreement (an expensive partial-refund guarantee) and with the clinic responsible for creating and storing our embryos. Among the questions we had to decide before my egg retrieval: what we would do with any unused embryos and what to do in case of divorce. I looked at our cost-share agreement recently and was surprised to find important details I don't remember reading or agreeing to—for example, that we would allow our doctor to transfer the number of embryos he thought best—but my signature is at the bottom of the page, right next to Richard's.

Compared with much of the world, we're exceedingly well equipped to evaluate contracts. Our ability to read and write, and the fact that any agreement we're expected to enter into is communicated to us in our native tongue, make us different from, for example, many of the surrogates who contract with agencies like Doron Mamet's. And still we overlooked things—not because we were cavalier or careless, but because we felt we had no other choice.

One of the paradoxes of Plan B family creation is that, despite the nonaccidental nature of the endeavor, the months and years of waiting and planning, the parties with the most at stake are often met by professionals who have a financial interest in moving things along. Adoptive parents-to-be are given minimal time to decide whether to retrieve a child from a hospital or orphanage; domestically, they are counseled to adopt in states that give birth mothers the smallest window of time for thinking about what it means to give up parental rights. ART patients are often not well informed at the beginning of the process about all of the medical and legal decisions they'll have to make on short notice. For LGBT parents-to-be, decisions made on the journey to parenthood are further complicated by a legal system that does not always recognize their rights, which can pressure them to accept whatever option is offered.

The only direct commentary from *Google Baby*'s director,

Zippi Brand Frank, comes at the beginning of the film, via epi-graph: "In the 60s, the introduction of the birth control pill took the risk of 'making babies' out of sex. Today, new technologies have taken sex out of the act of 'making babies.'" The absence of sex from the creation of life—test-tube babies stored in vats of liquid nitrogen—seems like old news to me. Instead, the most disturbing element of the film is the feeling that nothing is governed by rules and everything is rushed. Mamet counsels his clients over the phone or Skype and is surprised when three different couples agree to the suggestion, over the phone, that they transfer embryos to two surrogates at a time, increasing their odds of conception. In an IVF/OB clinic in Delhi, cesarean sections happen on screen in a matter of minutes, and the babies are whisked away after the briefest of glimpses from their surrogate mothers. "You're happy? Happy or not?" the obstetrician briskly asks a sedated woman who is silently weeping as the baby she carried is cleaned on a nearby table. The surrogate is not allowed even a moment of loss.

The imbalance of power inherent in the global surrogacy market is not merely a product of finances—the fact that surrogacy can be arranged in India, Mexico, or Nepal for about half what it would cost at home—but also of a confusing and often discriminatory legal landscape in the developed countries where the clients live. Israel has some LGBT-friendly laws and a profamily atmosphere that many same-sex couples find welcoming, but family law is decided by conservative rabbinical courts, and surrogacy for same-sex couples is a nonstarter. Ireland, which voted overwhelmingly to legalize same-sex marriage in 2015, forbids surrogacy and only recently began allowing adoption by same-sex couples. In the United States, the state-by-state landscape of surrogacy laws is varied and often unclear. And the fact that Gabe and Todd can't contract with a paid surrogate in their home state certainly increases the cost and inconvenience of surrogacy in California or Illinois.

So would-be parents are pushed into unregulated markets, where they enter into contracts with women whose greatest economic power resides in what their bodies can do—accept and grow an embryo from a few cells into a healthy baby.

"It would be completely disingenuous for anyone to suggest that the mercantile impulse isn't at play here," Gabe told me in an email. "But then again it's also at play—and in far more unregulated and even darker ways—with everything else Westerners buy through the globalized marketplace, which is to say almost literally everything."

Ideally, a younger friend would offer to take on Gabe and Todd's surrogacy. Briefly, I imagine myself as that heroic woman—what a gift that would be for two people I know will make excellent fathers. But then I think about timing (I'm nearing forty) and health risks and the all-consuming condition of *being pregnant,* and the situation starts to seem less cozy and altruistic than terrifying. Parul Goetz, who talked to me about her decision to adopt, considered surrogacy after her sister offered to carry her baby. But, she told me, "then I thought, I can't ask her to do that, and if I can't ask my own sister, how can I ask a stranger?"

That line of reasoning, informed by her own experiences with multiple pregnancies and miscarriages, led her to adopt domestically. For Gabe and Todd, the adoption of a newborn—asking a birth mother to give up her genetically related child—might be ethically more complicated than contractual surrogacy. I'm not sure I would have been comfortable with either choice, but then, I had an easier option available. Because I've been where Todd and Gabe are, where Nate and Parul once were—on the cusp of Plan B—I don't judge their choices. I can't.

It is now possible for almost anyone with resources to become a parent, through ART or other means. Couples strained by years of infertility can choose new treatment options, including preimplantation genetic screening of embryos or gene therapies that replace disease-carrying mitochondria with DNA from a third party. They can select donor eggs, sperm, or embryos. Single women and lesbians can choose from vast donor databases or opt for insemination from a known donor, in a clinic or at home, using a drugstore syringe. Couples and individuals can adopt domestically through private agencies or the foster-care system, or they can work with agencies and orphanages from all parts of the world. Gay men and lesbians or straight women can create unusual family arrangements through surrogacy and donor insemination agreements like the ones arranged by Solomon or Ertman, or they can combine one partner's sperm with donated eggs and have the embryos flown across the world to be gestated by a stranger.

The ever-expanding definition of *parenthood* is threatening to some, who emphasize the value of biological parenthood. But even the definition of *biological* has changed. We now know that every one of the parenting situations described above is biological, even at a genetic level, as the conditions we create as we raise children affect them right down to the expression of their DNA.

"The story of my life is constant evolution of identity," Gabe told me recently. "I'm constantly letting go of, or trying to let go of, the person I thought I was going to be."

This is also the story of marriage equality and reproductive equality—constant evolution, constant expansion. The use of reproductive technologies in expanding the public image of parenthood has been part of that evolving story. Martha Ertman wrote that she'd for a long time "wished that two eggs could make a baby, so that my lady love and I could have a child genetically linked to both of us." That was impossible, so she turned to reproductive technology; Ertman and her wife now represent one of the nearly 122,000 same-sex American households raising 210,000 American children.

But even as one reality (Plan B parenthood) supports another (same-sex marriage), and vice versa, our laws have not
caught up, and parents, children, and would-be parents are suffering. Adoption can still be more complicated, and more expensive, for same-sex couples, who may also experience bias
from adoption and foster-care agencies, particularly in states
allowing religious-liberty exemptions. Same-sex couples who
marry, perhaps in the hope of providing additional stability to
their children, or before starting a family through ART or other
means, can be fired from their jobs in more than half of the
United States. ART has been a frequent target of restriction,
whether through personhood amendments restricting IVF for
everyone or attempts to restrict IVF and ART to married heterosexual couples.

When I became a teacher, I was taught to differentiate my
instruction. Every lesson, every assessment, needed to consider not just the majority of the room but every student and
how she learned and expressed herself best. At first this felt
like an impossible task, time consuming and unnatural. I had to
create multiple sets of materials, give multiple kinds of home-
work and assessments, and it was difficult for me to imagine
what would work best for the students who weren't reached the
old-fashioned way. I'd been that kind of old-fashioned student,
content to sit in a chair, read from a textbook, and take traditional written tests (which was largely how my K–12 education
was conducted). But I tried to do what my education professors
asked, and I found that they were right: adapting my classroom
wasn't as hard as I feared, and it paid off. Everyone learned better this way—by expanding my instruction to meet the needs
of a few, I improved outcomes for all my students. A bonus: the
kids were happier.

Our legal system doesn't guarantee happiness (only its pursuit, ostensibly), but legislating inclusivity seems to work the
same way, at least where marriage and parenting are concerned.

"Pluralistic regulation better serves the purposes of family law," Douglas NeJaime told me. Which is? I asked. In part, NeJaime said, it's about "recognizing and supporting the various dependency relationships that we form, which often take the form of parent-child and spousal relationships—long supported by law—but increasingly take the form of other arrangements." When we regulate inclusively, we endeavor to protect everyone—children, same-sex couples, different-sex couples, donors, birth mothers, surrogates.

It's possible, after *Obergefell,* that North Carolina will consider the need to protect families that begin in surrogacy arrangements and will regulate accordingly. But for Gabe and Todd, who are ready to start their family now, that will be too late. Uncomfortable with the ethical uncertainties, the unknowns, they changed their minds about working with a foreign agency—fortunate timing, as the Nepali Supreme Court suspended that country's contractual surrogacy programs in late August 2015. Before the Nepal program's suspension, they'd consulted with Mamet as well as several different U.S.-based agencies and clinics. They're now hopeful about the possibility of contracting with an American surrogate—someone, Gabe says, with whom they could form a meaningful relationship.

I asked Gabe if he'd thought about what he and Todd will tell their potential child one day about the way he or she came into the world. "We'll be very up front with this kid," he said. He imagines telling the whole story once the child is old enough to understand, and also facilitating contact, at some point, with the egg donor and surrogate, if the women are open to that. "We'll also say, you are *our* child, because that's what we believe," Gabe told me.

Gabe and Todd celebrated their second wedding anniversary a couple of weeks before the Supreme Court decision was announced. Gabe remembered the many discussions they had with Rabbi Shalhevet, who performed their ceremony, about the practice and meaning of various Jewish rituals, which they adapted to suit their circumstances. They shortened the *hakafot,* in which the couple circles one another seven times, to three rotations each around the other and one final rotation around each other simultaneously. For the ritual glass stomping, which can symbolize the intended length of matrimony ("as long as it would take for someone to gather each and every tiny shard created by the broken glass and try to reassemble the thing perfectly and seamlessly—an eternity," Gabe explained), they used the more easily crushable lightbulb, as many modern couples do. Some rabbis don't consider a marriage complete until the couple spends a few minutes alone together in a private room known as a *yichud* before joining the wedding festivities. There was no *yichud* at the restaurant where they married, so Gabe and Todd walked around the block, "giddy and amazed and excited and moved" by what they'd done. This seems to me a metaphor not just for their marriage but also for their birth-story-to-be—adaptive but also rooted in tradition, privately decided but informed by a public context.

"What a journey it had been," Gabe said. "What a journey it continues to be."

Carrying

. . .

It was rainy and cold the day we transferred our embryo. A Sunday in late February, ordinarily the sort of day I'd spend feeling an acute teacher's dread of Monday—papers to grade, lessons to plan. But I'd taken the first part of the week off, and I remember coming home and lying down right away, not because I was tired or in pain but because I thought motionlessness would help our chances. The embryo had grown so well in the meticulously controlled laboratory environment, cells dividing evenly and on schedule. I tried to do the visualizations I'd read about—the embryo floating serenely in my uterine cavity, then attaching securely—but could not manage them and settled instead for stillness.

If attachment of one body to another is what defines a pregnancy, I was pregnant very early on Wednesday morning. I know because I felt it—a sharp pain, almost a twisting of my insides, that jolted me out of bed. I got up and walked around the house. The sky had cleared by then, and there was enough moonlight for me to find my way without turning on any lights. I walked until the pain dissipated, then climbed back under the covers.

The next morning my body had changed—my breasts were bigger, netted with blue veins, and tender. I lived tentatively in this new body for a day before asking a friend, going through her third IVF cycle then, if she thought you could see signs of pregnancy so soon. It was probably the progesterone suppositories we were both taking, she told me, a little apologetically and also, perhaps, a little bitterly. She must have felt or imagined the same signs in her previous cycles, both unsuccessful.

But by then I was sure. Every morning I told Richard, "I think I'm pregnant," and he said, "I think you are too." We bought a pregnancy test and decided I'd take it Sunday morning, one week after the transfer. I was so certain, I was hardly nervous waiting for the second line to turn pink. And there it was, definitive, in seconds. Later we went for a slow, ambling walk—it was warm, springlike, the banks of the Haw starting to green. We sat down in the new grass and watched an eagle make several passes in front of us before landing in her tree.

Our embarrassingly good luck: one IVF cycle yielding seven embryos, a second line on the pregnancy test that was even darker the next day, spring weather in early March. The first blood test I took at the clinic was definitive and reassuring. I returned two days later, expecting to find that the numbers had doubled. Instead my doctor called me with news he knew I'd find unsettling—they'd nearly quadrupled in two days, suggesting the possibility of twins. It wasn't unheard of, he told me, for a single embryo to become two, and we'd have to wait for the ultrasound to be sure.

My most reliable talent is an ability to find four-leaf clovers. I've found hundreds and hundreds of them, occasionally dozens at a time, and many favorite books in my house have browning flattened clovers tucked between random pages. My mother has this ability, too; you could say I inherited it from her, maybe a knack for spotting changes in pattern, but I think instead she taught me, by example, to look. I don't believe the clovers actually convey luck, but finding them calms me, buffers against anxiety, and maybe this confidence translates into good fortune

(conversely, not finding four-leaf clovers while actively search-
ing is alarming to me).

After getting the news that I might be carrying twins, I
made it my mission to find two four-leaf clovers every time I
walked to the river (the sunlight filtering along the river's leaf-
less edge apparently makes for ideal clover mutation, maybe
the Haw's history of pollution too). I pressed them into a small
black notebook, two at a time, page after page, until I didn't.

On March 25, Richard's birthday, I bled. It was dark out, and
we'd had dinner at home and were about to cut the cake I'd made
when the bleeding started. I was so shocked at the sight of all
that bright blood, I could barely register what it meant; Richard
called the doctor, who told us to come in the next morning for
an ultrasound. I was not six weeks pregnant yet; he wasn't sure
he'd be able to find a heartbeat. *Rest,* he told me. *There's nothing
anyone can do.*

We barely slept and the next morning drove silently to the
clinic, rode the elevator, and waited. Just weeks before we'd
carried in cookies for the staff, the hard stuff of injections and
retrieval behind us. But now I saw how we could easily be here
again, back at the beginning.

It was still too early for a regular ultrasound, the kind they
show on television. I put my feet in the stirrups and waited
for the transvaginal probing. The doctor, the same one I'd spoken to last night, was gentle and quiet. I held my breath. He
found the embryo—a single, tiny blob—and the clear *whish-
whish* of its heartbeat. He also discovered the source of my
bleeding: a large subchorionic hematoma, a bruise between the
placenta and the embryo. The hematoma could grow, ending
the pregnancy, or it could be absorbed by my body, the doctor
told us. *We'll just have to wait and see what happens,* he said.

He gave me a printout of the ultrasound image, and I thought
of weather maps and hurricanes, the fuzzed white space of at-
mospheric disturbances. I realized then that I was responding

not to the visual of the hematoma, a black blob that looked just like another cavity in my body, but of my own body's tissues, which appeared like static on the screen. The innocuous-looking bruise, which didn't even hurt, was in fact what threatened the embryo. By chance I saw our own doctor in the hallway and handed him the printout. It was a sizable hematoma, Dr. Young acknowledged. He reminded me that I was lucky to have the other frozen embryos.

But I didn't want those embryos—I wanted this one, which I'd already (against Richard's worried advice) read to and sung to, whose due date (November 19) I'd memorized. A perfect embryo, healthy and strong, with a heartbeat detectable before six weeks. How unfair that my body would fail it.

"It's always strange to me, the news of carrying, and how to hold it," wrote my friend the poet Elaine Bleakney when we communicated about my early pregnancy. I'd told her that the IVF was successful and then, a few weeks later, that I was scared and on a kind of modified, mostly self-prescribed bed rest: walking slowly from my bed to the living room, where I ate clementines, sent emails, and tried to write. During this time I had weekly ultrasounds and watched the hematoma shrink but not disappear, while the embryo—by then we'd seen it wriggle, froglike—grew steadily.

How to hold it: there is a reason it's common to keep pregnancy news a secret until the second trimester. We want to save ourselves, and our friends and family, the heartbreak of bad news delivered quickly on the heels of good. But in an IVF cycle, if you tell anyone what you're up to, you'll be asked how it went; you're also so used to constant updates and monitoring that it becomes all you think about.

At least, it was for me. I moved slowly, alert to stray twinges and phantom pains, and took up vigorous daily walks again only after the hematoma was gone, around the end of my first trimester. I drank not a drop of alcohol; I switched to decaf coffee. I had our water tested and bought bottled water after the results came back high for manganese. I ate meat for the first time in twenty years, slept only on my left side, did kick counts twice a day. I filled the rest of my bound, black book with four-leaf clovers.

Halfway through the pregnancy, I went on a kayaking trip with Richard and a friend; it stormed, and we pulled our boats to the shore and sat on the banks in pouring rain until the lightning and thunder stopped. But it just kept raining, and the river was so full, there was no turning back, nothing to do but paddle to the next landing. About a mile from our destination, we hit turbulent rapids and capsized. A stray tree branch scratched the side of my face as I fell, ripping a stud earring out of my ear. I swam back to my boat and pushed it to an island that divided the river. On either side of the island, the normally gently riffled water looked like ocean waves, and I could picture falling again, hitting my head, tumbling, scraping bottom, drowning. All I could think, when we finally climbed out of the river, was how foolish I'd been, and I held my stomach until I could feel again the reassuring kicks.

Those were the two major events of my pregnancy—some bleeding, and falling out of a boat in rushing water. Other than the fact that I never went to the bathroom without fear of seeing blood, the rest was routine. We found out the baby's sex at twenty weeks—both of us overjoyed to expect a girl—and took a childbirth-preparation class at the hospital where we used to go for fertility treatment. The doula who taught the class talked a lot about "normal birth" and the importance of resisting pitocin and epidurals during labor. The idea was that once you gave in to a medicalized birth experience, you'd never regain your control. You wouldn't be able to walk around or squat on a birthing ball or do any of the exercises we practiced in class.

I found her concept of normal birth alienating—not just her

suggestion that we would have to fight with the doctors to maintain our control, but also the idea that pregnancy and childbirth are normal and natural. "Your bodies know what to do," she told us. She showed us videos of normal hospital births and normal home births, and of a newborn crawling agonizingly slowly—no assistance needed—across her mother's stomach to reach her breasts. When someone in class asked our teacher how to do the rhythmic breathing we'd all seen in movie labor scenes, she scoffed and did a quick and disturbing pantomime. "Who doesn't know how to *breathe*?"

Who can't do what her body knows how to do?

What does the body know anyway?

Someone in the room's afraid. Kristen and Mara reading each other and Paul and then I'm pathetic. Then hope. Then another dim revolting wave.

I can't animal I tell Kristen when she's an eye. She knows he's lodged. I don't know or leave it says the tide. She's reading me stay here okay.

That's a passage from Elaine's collection of prose poetry, *For Another Writing Back,* describing the midwife-assisted home birth of her son, which happened in her Fort Greene apartment. I love Elaine's whole stunning book, which she began a few years after we were in graduate school together, but I have read the birth scenes over and over again. I love her intense, intimate descriptions of powerlessness, of going to the animal place of pain and pushing. I heard her read from this poem and watched an audience of listeners hold their breath until she got to the birth: *We're this? Then tucked on me his mouth he's so. He's so.*

Richard and I entered the hospital very early on November 23, not long after my water broke at home. The first question the nurse in the maternity triage room asked me, prone and having contractions on the examination table, was whether I'd thought about the kind of birth control I planned to use after the baby was born. "The pill?" I offered.

I wasn't afraid, but time moved in a fractured way, split, as the birthing-class instructor warned, by the various levels of medical intervention presented and accepted. "They call it labor and delivery, not rest and delivery," the pip-squeak male resident admonished me in the morning, when I refused pitocin and my contractions weren't any stronger. By noon, tired of walking the dull hallways and worried by the doctors' insistence, I agreed: pitocin, but only a little, an impossible request. My nurse kept turning it up, and up, and up, punching numbers into the IV machine next to my bed in what felt to me like a violent and sneaky way. I can't recall what my pitocin-augmented contractions felt like, not the way I can recollect the specific pain of a burn or a cut. I remember thinking they felt metallic, and I no longer had any desire to walk.

The hospital offered a volunteer doula program, and we summoned one doula, a young woman who finally showed me, crouching in the bathtub, how to breathe through the pain. That woman had to leave, and she called in two more doulas, new to the volunteer program. They were kind but no match for the nurse, punching up my pitocin on the half hour.

Around midnight I'd had enough. "Thank you, doulas, but I need an epidural," I said. Or I said something similar. No heroics for me—I never got to the place where Elaine went, waves of hot pain, a failure of language. Richard remembers that my voice was eerily calm when I woke him from a brief nap. "It's time," I told him. "The baby's coming."

The nurse who'd turned up the pitocin held one leg, Richard the other. A doctor in cowboy boots, also newly awakened, was quickly gowned and gloved. I pushed when she told me, as hard as I could, though I could barely feel what I was doing, as if by decisive pushing I could make up for my low pain threshold. "Do you want to catch the baby?" the doctor asked Richard. He hesitated and then said yes. "Wait," I said. But it was time to push again. Did I want to see her head?

Then there she was, in Richard's startled arms: squalling, pink, alert, round-cheeked, blue-eyed, ten-fingered, ten-toed, ours.

Later I wrote an abbreviated birth story in Beatrice's baby book, where I pasted some of the four-leaf clovers I'd found for her, which had all gone brittle and gray-green. The writing has the tone of a children's story ("It took a while," I wrote about my twenty-six-hour labor. ". . ."), though now I imagine she'll read the book when she's older, a teenager or an adult. I have all the ultrasounds tucked in the back of the book—the very first one, before the transfer; the ones after the hematoma. I'm not sure what to do with them, these early glimpses of her life, earlier than almost anyone has a chance to see. Perhaps they won't mean much to her; maybe she won't give them more than a passing glance.

Of course she'll know how dearly she was wanted by her parents, how long awaited, how precious. But I hope she'll also know how many other people—the doctors, nurses, embryologists, and general well-wishers—were there too, rooting for her, for us. If she thinks at all about chance and luck, longtime preoccupations of her mother, I hope she thinks not of the fragility of life, but its bounty.

Paying for It

• • •

"I wouldn't have this child without Massachusetts insurance," my friend Margaret Monteith told me over Skype one December morning. She was talking about the baby she expected in May, a somersaulting boy recently glimpsed, at the end of her first trimester, on ultrasound. It had taken Margaret and her husband, Matthew, nine rounds of IVF, seven miscarriages, and extraordinary patience and self-advocacy to achieve this pregnancy. At sixteen weeks along, Margaret was happily nesting and had just converted a small back bedroom of her Jamaica Plain apartment into a guest room for visiting family and friends. She'd checked out day cares and preschools; she'd been reading books on sleep schedules. She turned her computer screen so that I could see the spindled antique crib, a family heirloom dating to the 1800s, already set up in the corner of her living room.

Margaret is a writer and middle school teacher; she loves running and the outdoors and looks to my eyes a decade younger than her age of forty-five. We met in 2011 at a summer conference for writers, talked books and stories, gossiped, drank wine, went swimming, commiserated about K–12 teaching and the writing life; but the greatest sorrow of both our lives—that we could not have children without prohibitively expensive medical treatment—never once came up. At the time, she and her husband, a photographer and college professor, lived in

New York; what they earned that did not go to rent, food, utilities, and student loan payments went to premiums on a health insurance plan that would never cover the comprehensive fertility treatment they needed.

Margaret was thirty-seven when she began trying to get pregnant, thirty-eight when she first saw a reproductive endocrinologist. "My ob-gyn never indicated any problems at any point in my life before I began trying and it didn't work, so while I was aware that infertility is always a possibility, I wasn't too worried, just aware of the possibility based on friends' experiences," she said. "I wasn't worried about my age either, as my ob-gyn wasn't, the first RE I went to wasn't, and so many of my friends are older mothers."

Like me, Margaret tried less-expensive treatments first: oral medication, intrauterine insemination. These treatments are so much less effective than IVF that most clinics don't even keep careful track of them; doctors seem to be guessing when they offer success rates. "Ten percent? Fifteen?" It wasn't until a lucky break—new jobs for Margaret and her husband in Boston—that more aggressive treatment became an option. By then she was forty-two.

New York, where Margaret and her husband lived when they first sought treatment, is one of fifteen states requiring some coverage for infertility treatment in all insurance plans written for its residents. The problem for people like Margaret is that coverage is mandated only for "the diagnosis and treatment of a correctable medical condition, solely because the condition results in infertility." That means that a woman with a correctable tubal blockage, or a man with a varicocele affecting sperm production, could have surgery to correct those issues, even though surgery might not be the most effective or fastest treatment, and even though those issues are less common, for example, than diminished ovarian reserve or poor sperm count. IVF—often the most effective treatment, and the one most people have trouble affording—is specifically excluded from New York's mandate.

Reading about the mandatory coverage requirements of the fourteen other states is like looking at a map meant to show arbitrary signs of regional diversity: this state calls soft drinks pop, this one Coke. Arkansas, for example, allows for IVF treatment—but only up to a lifetime maximum of $15,000. Maryland insurance plans pay for IVF, but only with "the patient's eggs" and "her spouse's sperm." Rhode Island insurers provide up to $100,000 to "presumably healthy married individuals" who are forty years old or younger. Hawaii provides for a single IVF cycle, but only after a couple really tries: its plans require five years of infertility. Montana and West Virginia require coverage for infertility without defining the condition or the amount or type of coverage. By contrast, Illinois appears quite generous, requiring plans to pay for up to six egg retrievals—until you look more closely and see that only someone successful after four retrievals (experiencing a "live birth") may return for the other two.

It's easy to see, even in states that have attempted to provide infertility coverage, who gets left out: people who have complicated diagnoses or need expensive treatment, like Margaret; people who are older; LGBT couples, people in unmarried partnerships, or women who have decided to get pregnant on their own. "I have friends who live elsewhere who don't have this level of insurance and don't make enough money to pay for the treatments. Many of my friends who have been able to afford it either had high paying jobs or well-off parents to help them," Margaret told me. "It's heartbreaking to me because it seems that having children should not be based on being wealthy enough."

In the RESOLVE support group I attended for more than two years, we rarely talked about money or the cost of treatment. Someone might mention that her health insurance covered IVF or injectable meds, or describe a package plan purchased through one of the local clinics, but the people who gathered around the hospital basement table were as different in terms of what we paid for care as the random collection of states with IVF coverage were in terms of what they covered. More than that, the connection between our financial circumstances and our ability to achieve and sustain a pregnancy was too great, and too sensitive. More than any other factor—age, sperm count and quality, egg reserve as measured by hormonal tests—the resources we could allocate to treatment appeared to determine our outcomes. It was a numbers game, I began to believe as I saw, again and again, the most intrepid injectors and IVFers and IUIers finally dropping out of our group: they were pregnant, at long last.

Not everyone achieved her pregnancy the same way: one woman in my group injected the last of her follicle-stimulating medication, left over from a previous cycle, without telling her husband; they had sex and she became pregnant with twins. Another woman, after failing at IVF and countless cycles with injectable medication and timed sex, went back to IUIs and conceived her daughter. One couple tried embryo adoption, another donor egg, and both went on to have healthy pregnancies. I remember thinking that some of these women should give up, move on—they'd had so many failures, so many interventions, they'd never get pregnant.

A few did just that; they'd exhausted their resources after one or two cycles of IVF and could no longer bear the way meetings reminded them of their failures. But of those of us who could afford all the costs that many rounds of medical treatment entail—the drain on savings or credit, the emotional turmoil, the time away from work—all became pregnant, one by one returning to the group to announce the shockingly good news. It was the reverse of the ill-considered folk wisdom most of us had heard from family or friends: *As soon as you stop trying, you'll get pregnant.* Our truth was more like this: *Keep trying*—an expensive proposition for almost all of us—*and you'll eventually have success.*

The biggest difference I noticed at our fertility clinic's new suburban location, aside from nicer waiting and examination rooms, was in how we made our payments. While we once wrote checks and processed insurance claims through UNC Fertility, now all financial interactions would go through IntegraMed, a company that runs niche outpatient medical centers ("dominant," according to their website, in fertility and vein clinics).

We knew this and had already paid IntegraMed $20,200, just a few days after returning from Iceland. In exchange for the overwhelmingly large bank draft, we received a contract eight pages long, detailing a strange financial arrangement known euphemistically as a cost-share plan. According to our contract, the money we paid made us eligible for up to three rounds of IVF and three frozen-embryo transfers. The arrangement didn't cover medications, but the most expensive IVF line items—the egg retrieval and fertilization, the embryo culturing, the transfer—would be paid for ahead of time, in a lump sum that allowed us, as the brochures promised, to "focus on having a baby!"

Behind IntegraMed's cheery messaging—their fertility-related website exhorts patients to "plan for success" and offers a chatty, inspirational blog—Richard recognized something else. Without the option of insurance—our state was not among those with even vague requirements—we'd hedged our bets, buying into something closer to a financial derivative, such as a credit default swap, than a health insurance plan.

A credit default swap works like this: One party wants to sell an asset with an uncertain future value—for example, a pool of mortgages with an average interest rate of 7 percent—for a flat price in the present. The buyer manages her risk by requiring additional security from the seller: if those mortgages don't return at 7 percent—if a significant group of homeowners defaults and they pay out at only 3 percent, for example—the seller agrees to cover part of the buyer's loss. The product is often nothing as specific or tangible as a mortgage; it's just a bunch of money, an opportunity, a bet.

Had we paid for IVF treatment per cycle, we would have been charged approximately $11,000 for each cycle. It was likely that I'd need more than one cycle to get pregnant—in fact, I might need all three, and it was easy to imagine losing our nerve after the first or second failure. And what if three, or even four or five, cycles failed? Under a traditional payment arrangement, we'd be out tens of thousands of dollars, some of it borrowed or liquidated from our retirement plans. With the cost-share plan, we'd get a 70 percent refund if we did not "take home a baby," money we imagined reinvesting into adoption or foster-care expenses.

We were betting, then, on our own failure—just one failed cycle would make the plan financially sound. IntegraMed was betting on our success. They'd verified my age (thirty-six at entry to the program), the level of my hormones indicating my egg reserve, and the results of Richard's sperm analysis; they'd reviewed a hydrosonogram to check the condition of my uterus. I was healthy, and my ovarian reserve qualified me for the program, though the contract I signed stipulated that IntegraMed could cancel my participation and provide a refund for "any reason in its reasonable discretion": if my ovaries didn't produce enough retrievable eggs, if the embryos were of poor quality, if I suddenly gained or lost a lot of weight, had a bad reaction to medication, ignored medical advice, or passed my thirty-eighth birthday.

Looking back, it's easy to see that the deal was always skewed in their favor. IntegraMed could cancel our contract at any time, provided they refunded 70 percent of our money—they have many clients and, presumably, extensive actuarial data to consult when considering the best time to back out. A friend from my support group was surprised and distraught to have her IntegraMed contract terminated after two cycles; she thought she'd get at least three chances, as the brochures and website suggest. Still, she didn't think of the arrangement as a bad deal—with 70 percent of her money returned, she could afford to try again at another clinic.

Richard and I knew that spending more money than we would have under a traditional payment arrangement was a possibility; that was the possibility we hoped for, in fact. We hoped to spend more money than we needed, hoped that our precaution—all those extra cycles, fresh and frozen—would prove overzealous. The website that advertised our package plan promoted it as a way of controlling costs, managing stress, and removing the unknown from our treatment plan. In some guilt-prone, superstitious part of my brain, I must have thought, too, that paying more might make me worthier of success. Perhaps by paying extra I could skip the miscarriages, chemical pregnancies, cancelled cycles, and laparoscopic surgeries of my peers—those offerings of suffering I'd seen so many others make on the journey to parenthood.

When I became pregnant from our first cycle, I didn't regret the money we spent or wish we'd chosen differently. After dreading IVF, hating the nightly injections as much as I expected, and desperately fearing a poor outcome, I was relieved and joyous, taking not one but three pregnancy tests, just to watch the second line turn pink again. I didn't think about the $9,000 we might have saved for other health-care costs—our daughter's birth, for example—or expenses associated with having a family. Regret didn't enter my mind.

I refused to think of the money, in fact, for the duration of my pregnancy, fearing that to do so would be ungrateful, greedy, a tempting of fate. Now, when I think back on the financial arrangement we entered into with IntegraMed, I am of two minds: happy that we made the decision but sorry that we had so few other choices. Further, I'm troubled by the idea that investors are somewhere making money by exploiting the lack of coverage for a financially and emotionally risky medical procedure.

My happiness with the decision is of course bolstered by the conception and birth of my daughter—how could I feel any other way? But I'm far enough removed from the experience of IVF—she's crawling toward me as I write this—to know that I would have been just as likely to get pregnant had I paid less.

I believe that my pregnancy was safer because of the cost-share program, however, and this is the primary reason I'd make the same choice if I had to do it again.

Patients undergoing IVF are hoping, generally, for high numbers: we want to retrieve as many mature eggs as possible, and for those eggs to fertilize and develop into multiple embryos. A greater number of embryos means that doctors can select the best, most regularly celled and advanced for transfer. On day three of the embryos' development, embryologists like to see embryos with six, seven, eight, or nine regular cells.

We were lucky to have a number of embryos available to transfer—ten on day three, with seven developing to the blastocyst stage on day five. Years earlier, when our doctor first suggested IVF, I remember Richard joking, "Twins would be fine!" Dr. Young cautioned, reasonably, that his goal was for his patients to have one healthy baby at a time, and by now we agreed. I'd read about the health risks for twins, including prematurity, low birth weight, an increased chance of prescribed bed rest for me—the best way to avoid this, I knew, was to transfer a single embryo.

I'm not sure how many of Dr. Young's patients purchase a cost-share plan, as we did—the clinic doesn't advertise or publish that information—but I believe that anticipating a financially mitigated failure (we would be responsible for medication but not the cost of another transfer or IVF cycle) gave us the confidence to choose a single embryo transfer. SET is commonly practiced in European countries with mandated IVF coverage—in Sweden, for example, 70 percent of all IVF procedures are elective single embryo transfer, and the twin rate from IVF is 5 percent (by contrast, our clinic's twin rate for my age group was around 30 percent).

Responsible doctors like ours routinely mention the risks associated with twin births while misunderstanding some of the financial motivations behind their patients' choices. In a blog post for his clinic, Reproductive Medicine Associates of New Jersey, Dr. Thomas Molinaro blamed our success-driven culture: "In America we are consumers and we are inundated every day with the consumer mentality," he wrote.

There is no doubt that everybody wants to be successful and they want the best chance at pregnancy. But sometimes patients view themselves as a customer purchasing a product rather than as a patient coming to a physician for treatment. The biggest obstacle I face to single embryo transfer is the couple sitting across the table from me who are weighing the risk of a twin pregnancy with the potential improvement in success. Time and time again I hear patients say that they would rather have two embryos transferred because it improves success and they just can't bear the thought of another negative pregnancy test.

New Jersey, where Dr. Molinaro works, has one of the most generous IVF mandates, requiring insurance companies to pay for up to four IVF retrievals. In fact, his clinic boasts a 30 percent SET rate for women in my age group—more than three times higher than the national average and six times higher than the one at my clinic. But Dr. Molinaro's hesitant patients may anticipate needing more than four cycles, or they may work at a small company or for a religious employer—both are excluded from New Jersey's mandate.

Because Richard and I spent two years saving for IVF, we were able to fake a limited kind of insurance coverage through the purchase of an unregulated financial derivative, insulating us against the kind of risky decision making that is routine in most clinics. On the day of transfer, our doctor and embryologist showed us two embryos—the one they'd chosen, already hatching, and the runner-up, which might have accompanied the first. *You have about a fifty-fifty chance,* Dr. Young told us, *slightly higher if you go with two.* I was in a hospital gown and socks, my abdomen still swollen and sore from the retrieval days before. I held the photos of the embryos in my hands, ours to keep. We hesitated, just for a moment, before sticking by our decision. Five weeks later, we saw the heartbeat.

Just one, as we'd hoped.

We told Richard's parents about the pregnancy at a Chinese restaurant in March. We hadn't told them that we were pursuing IVF, though they knew we'd been in treatment for infertility for years. After exclaiming in joy and praying aloud, Richard's mother asked us the first question that came to her mind: "Did you do it the natural way, or did you pay eighty thousand dollars?"

"Neither," Richard said firmly. He explained the IVF process to his parents without telling them how much we'd spent or how we'd saved the money.

I'm not sure if $80,000 represented a real amount Richard's mother imagined us capable of spending, or hyperbole meant to express the exorbitant price of assisted reproduction. Eighty thousand dollars was more than Richard's family paid for their first house, more than my parents paid for the house they live in now. It was also, of course, significantly more than we paid for our IVF package and medication. But it's not an impossible number with tough cases—Margaret Monteith's three-year odyssey would have cost far more than that had she paid entirely out of pocket (even with Massachusetts's comparatively generous insurance plan, treatment wiped out Margaret and her husband's savings). Maybe my mother-in-law had heard how much some celebrity paid for their miracle baby, or read an article about cases like Margaret's.

More interesting to me is the way that great sum of money represented, for my mother-in-law, the most salient feature of my unnatural pregnancy. What was most unnatural and confusing about it was not the way it had been accomplished—outside of the womb, in a laboratory—but the fact that we'd paid for it to happen.

Surgeries and serious medical treatments often cost more than most of us can comfortably imagine. I asked my mother the cost of my father's major surgeries—a triple heart bypass, followed by surgery to repair an aortic abdominal aneurysm. "Oh, a million dollars," she told me. "At least." She didn't know an exact number because insurance paid for most of it and the staggering total was spread out over a series of bills delivered weeks and months after the fact, tallying the portions paid by insurance to each provider. Even if they'd had no insurance, he would have been able to have the surgeries—their necessity would have trumped any assessment of whether my parents could pay. I'm pretty sure that no one has ever asked him, *Did you stay alive the natural way, or did you spend a million dollars?*

IVF is an elective procedure with a poor success rate and an arguably unnecessary goal. But it is also true that infertility is an emotionally punishing experience as well as a disability, which qualifies workers for some protection under the Americans with Disabilities Act. It's hard to imagine that the stress of infertility isn't compounded by the question of how to pay for treatment, so much that, almost against our wills, it crowds out other thinking. Like my mother-in-law, we think in trade-offs: Will I put a down payment on a house or maybe have a baby? Will I max out these credit cards? Liquidate this retirement plan? Take out a second mortgage?

In his semi-autobiographical novel *10:04,* Ben Lerner writes about a poet-turned-novelist with the surprising good fortune of a "strong six figure" deal for an unwritten new novel, who is also undergoing assisted reproduction with his best friend. At a celebratory dinner with his agent, Lerner's narrator is bewildered by the large advance, an amount that feels both abstract and spoken for, thanks to his uncertain personal circumstances. "Imitative desire for my virtual novel was going to fund artificial insemination and its associated costs . . . ," he considers. "I would clear something like two hundred and seventy thousand dollars. Or Fifty-four IUIs. Or around four Hummer H2 SUVs. Or the two first editions on the market of *Leaves of Grass.*"

In my support group, though we didn't talk about the specific price tags of our treatments, some of us would occasionally mention what we exchanged for the opportunity to try them: vacations we didn't take, down payments on houses we didn't buy. Some of us stayed in jobs we hated, just to keep our health insurance. Like Lerner's narrator, we converted windfalls—those of us lucky enough to experience them—into treatments. Some of us thought of moving to places with better insurance laws, a prospect complicated by a bad economy and the various demands of our careers. We traveled out of state, to adoption conferences and clinical studies, researched the cost of "vacation IVF" in Mexico or Europe, and bought discounted, leftover meds online. We were always looking for a bargain, always thinking of the money, not because we were necessarily money-minded people but because we had no other choice.

Swept up in the excitement of their new jobs, Margaret and her husband didn't realize the greatest benefit of their New York–to–Boston move until Margaret spoke to a friend who'd also gone through ART in New York. "His first response was, 'Great! Do you know they cover IVF in Massachusetts?'" Margaret told me. She did some research and called her new insurance company, just to verify things, as soon as she received her policy. Unaffordable out-of-pocket expenses in New York became manageable copays in Boston. "It was an enormous relief to learn that we could do it, that insurance would cover much of the costs. It feels great to live in a state where not only infertility treatments are covered, but also one where everyone has access to basic health insurance and health care, period."

Still, Margaret's treatment wasn't easy. Because she had waited so long—she was forty-two when she first saw her Boston RE and began IVF—her doctors believed that her recurrent miscarriages were related to her age and egg quality. They strongly recommended using donor eggs, and Margaret and her husband took their advice, which involved more out-of-pocket expenses, more waiting. When those cycles, too, ended in miscarriage, Margaret finally persuaded her doctors to investigate her thyroid and autoimmune issues. Her doctors researched expensive new supplemental medications to try, including an injection that would have cost $7,000 without insurance (it was covered); they planned a cycle, using previously frozen embryos, with these drugs.

"At our planning meeting, my doctor kept referring to the left-over embryos," she said. "And I said, what about *my* embryos?"

Margaret and her husband had two frozen embryos left over from their very first IVF cycle in Boston, when she was forty-two, as well as several from a donor cycle. On paper, her cycles had always gone better than her twenty-two-year-old donor's—she produced more eggs, and the resulting embryos were more numerous and of a higher quality. The doctor agreed to compare the donor-cycle and traditional IVF embryos and reported back that the ones from Margaret's cycle were in fact more advanced—they had seven and nine cells, while the donor-egg embryos were all four celled. He was still skeptical.

"The doctor said, 'It's up to you,'" Margaret said. "To be honest I don't think he thought it would work." Margaret and her husband chose to transfer the embryos created with Margaret's eggs; they went in to the clinic on a warm September morning, then to a friend's book launch that night. During the two weeks of waiting they took walks on the beach, watched the sunset, ate lobster. "I felt cautiously optimistic about our chances on transfer day and during the waiting period because I felt like they had finally addressed the medical issues," she told me. "It all went well that day, but I don't remember so much of that day versus other ones because at this point, I have had so many transfers. I do remember feeling slightly less anxious about it all, maybe because I'd been through it so many times and because I felt, instinctually, that the protocol was finally right." Her singleton pregnancy was confirmed later that month; a few weeks later she saw the baby on ultrasound. "He flipped!" she remembered. "It was one of the most exciting and happy things I've ever seen."

To hear this news from Margaret was a great, unexpected lift. I'd stopped emailing her regularly after writing to her about my pregnancy, which happened when she was forty-three, just after her doctor persuaded her to move on to donor eggs. At the time she was diligently working on the attendant paperwork: screening candidates, dealing with attorneys' fees and other headaches. Margaret seemed genuinely happy, even elated, for me, but every time I thought about checking in with her after that, I hesitated. Most women I know in infertility circles cheer each other on—it's encouraging to see other people succeed, especially the tough or long-standing cases—but it can be hard to watch someone progress through pregnancy and childbirth while you wait: for treatments to work, for endometriosis to resolve or a cyst to be removed, for the financial or emotional means to try again. For a pregnant woman, nine months can seem endlessly long, but in infertility treatment, it goes by in a flash—*Nine more months,* you think: *I should be pregnant by now. I thought I'd have a baby.*

In my own support group, the custom after getting pregnant was to go to one last meeting to let people know—there would be exclamations, tears, sometimes hugs—and then never return. I knew a kind, funny woman who left our group in despair after two failed, expensive IVFs; I was able to keep up with her on Facebook, but after a while her posts disappeared. Another friend from the group told me the reason: she'd unfriended us, one by one, as we got pregnant. "I don't blame her," my other friend said. "I'd have done the same thing."

Margaret was different, though: she emailed me every few months, even as her journey seemed all uphill, mine all downhill. She asked after my health when I was on bed rest and sent well wishes on my birthday (I am a terrible birthday rememberer). Possibly this is just the sort of person she is—a writer used to the long and lonely work of novel writing, a teacher used to looking after others, an artist accustomed to the many disappointments on the way to her big break. Maybe it was the care she was taking in her health, running and walking miles every day, or the benefits of acupuncture treatment and meditation. Maybe it's genetic.

But I suspect that there was something more to Margaret's equanimity and fortitude, something related to the structural protection in her state's insurance laws. Virtually everyone in Massachusetts has health care—the coverage level today is at 99 percent, the highest in the nation. And, according to law, insurers must provide for artificial insemination; for IVF and intracytoplasmic sperm injection (ICSI); and for donor sperm, egg, or embryo procurement and processing. Medication coverage is handled just like medication for any other health problem. There is no limit to the number of treatment cycles and no cap on expenditures. Infertility patients in Margaret's state don't begin their treatment afraid it might bankrupt them or make other options—adoption or foster care, for example— impossible; they begin committed to the long haul. Perhaps most significantly, they begin knowing that they will be treated, at least in the eyes of their insurance, like any other patient with any other medical condition.

Barbara Collura, who as the president and CEO of RESOLVE has spent more than ten years strategizing and advocating for better health insurance mandates, put it this way: "Patients make better health decisions when the issue of finances isn't hanging over their heads."

That was true for us, though the amount we spent to make those decisions would have been unaffordable for most, and though the financial anvil was only slightly off to the side— maybe not over our heads, but over our shoulders or our feet, or some other important body part. IntegraMed and their investors made money from our bet, but I remain convinced that making it is one reason I gave birth at almost forty-one weeks to a healthy baby.

Still, I wonder what my support group might have been like if we all had health insurance we couldn't lose and the ability to keep going when treatments failed. Would we have been more open? Less afraid, less anxious, less tearful? Would the group have gotten smaller more quickly, as people moved into the treatments with the best chances of success? Freed from financial worry, would I have gone at all?

Margaret, who did not attend a support group in all her eight years of infertility, wonders something else: "What if men were the ones having babies? Would we pay for treatment then?"

In a 2012 study of advertising by fertility clinics, law professor Jim Hawkins examined the websites of 372 clinics listed by the Society for Assisted Reproductive Technology (SART), a voluntary-membership organization that reports success rates for 90 percent of IVF clinics in the United States. Hawkins found that clinics emphasized the emotional rather than the practical side of fertility treatment: 79 percent of the clinics featured photographs of babies on their home pages, 30 percent used the word *dream* on the home page, and 8.87 percent used the word *miracle*. Although Hawkins notes that "price is usually one of the most important terms in a consumer transaction," he found that only 27 percent of websites listed any kind of pricing for IVF. After suggesting a number of possible reasons—the aversion many doctors have to talking price with patients, the difficulty of predicting the cost of treatment, or an assumption that patients aren't cost driven—Hawkins concludes that "it seems more likely that clinics are purposefully refusing to present price information to focus patients' attention away from price."

Hawkins doesn't draw this distinction, but I wonder if clinics are also making assumptions based on a narrow target audience: women, specifically educated, older, white, upper-middle-class women. Though we know that infertility affects men as often as women (30 percent of infertility cases are attributable to male infertility, 30 percent to female, with 40 percent a combination or unexplained), women are more likely to research clinics and make the first appointment. Perhaps clinics imagine themselves marketing to women driven by fantasy and emotion, women swayed by soft-focus images of mothers and babies, uninterested in thinking of IVF as a highly uncertain consumer transaction. (To the contrary, I remember a professional, impeccably dressed fortyish woman in my support group who, faced with an unpromising-looking group of embryos, casually remarked that she was "playing with the B team.")

The stereotypical image of an infertility patient is itself a fantasy. Infertility is not only as likely to be a male problem as it is a female one, but it is also more likely to affect minorities, the poor, and the less educated. Although SART has established guidelines for more accurate and transparent advertising, Hawkins found a low level of compliance among its membership. Clinics not only hid treatment costs and success rates, but they tended to focus their marketing more heavily on white patients. More than 97 percent of clinics included photographs of white babies on their websites, and 62 percent featured only photographs of white babies. Hawkins speculated that skewed advertising could attract white patients while driving away minorities. More disturbing, he noted that "it is possible that clinics are purposefully using the race of babies to draw in white patients, confirming the charge of some academics who argue that fertility treatments entrench racist norms."

And the doctors themselves are vulnerable to misconceptions. A 2010 study of physician perceptions of infertility revealed that few understood the major risk factors—only 16 percent of the physicians surveyed correctly identified African Americans as the most at risk for infertility, and an even smaller percentage, 13 percent, recognized that women without high school diplomas are more likely to be infertile than women with higher educational attainment. Instead, the surveyed doctors' perceptions tended to match stereotypes about fertility patients, familiar from movies, television, and IVF advertising. Even scientific studies of infertility tend to focus on this limited demographic group.

In the United States, infertility affects one in eight couples, but only half of those affected seek medical treatment; those who do tend to be white, older, wealthy, and educated. Demographics can expand when coverage is financially accessible to everyone—a 2013 Canadian study, conducted after Quebec mandated IVF insurance coverage, showed that removing financial barriers increased both socioeconomic and racial diversity. But in the United States, a variety of conflicting studies have indicated that cost is not the only barrier. Massachusetts's insurance mandate, for example, allowed Margaret to conceive her son, but minorities and patients with lower incomes and educational attainment are still underrepresented within that state. One study of Massachusetts women treated with IVF postmandate showed that 85 percent of its subjects had at least a college degree, while none had less than a high school diploma.

Some barriers are more nuanced. Maybe you have Medicaid and your doctor doesn't think you'll be able to afford the treatment you need, so she doesn't refer you to a specialist. Maybe you don't feel comfortable talking to your doctor—what if you speak a different language than she does or you can't read the medical literature she has available? Maybe you don't see a physician for preventative care. If you do manage a referral, the RE clinic might seem inaccessible for other reasons—too far from where you live, with inconvenient hours and no mention of price on its website, only images of people who don't look like you or the baby you imagine.

"Medicine serves as a gatekeeper," writes sociologist Ann V. Bell in a study of inequality of access. By focusing research on women already accessing treatment and ignoring the diverse, day-to-day life experiences of women who live with infertility, the medical establishment reinforces racist and classist norms, Bell claims, and risks "determining who should and should not mother."

Bell argues that the rise of ART and the subsequent medicalization of infertility has made childlessness more deviant and other avenues to motherhood less desirable. As part of her study, she interviewed twenty-seven Michigan-based women of low socioeconomic status who had been trying to conceive for more than a year. The women noted a number of barriers and approaches to IVF treatment that are familiar to me, even as my hurdles were more easily cleared. With no insurance coverage and little time off from work to attend midday appointments, they were always making plans and revising strategies—maybe they'd sell their cars, move out of state, or make peace with their conditions. But these strategies and decisions were devised very much on their own—many reported that they never felt a doctor wanted to help them become mothers. Some turned to folk medicine, rubbing pregnant stomachs for luck, or making wishes:

> *When I held [a friend's] baby the first time . . . I thought— because I—I—I just loved her up and I thought, "I want one of these, I want one of these." It was like wishing on a star or something, you know.*

There are people working to break down these barriers at institutional and grassroots levels. RESOLVE provides training to volunteers who want to start free, peer-led support groups; there are now more than two hundred groups in forty-six states, plus the District of Columbia. Online communities of infertile and TTC women are not only numerous, but warm and inclusive. Other organizations, such as Fertility for Colored Girls or the Broken Brown Egg, host both online communities and in-person events designed to increase awareness about infertility in minority communities. They help provide a safe and supportive place to find out about treatment and other resources, or just to express sadness or frustration.

"I try to just say and address all of the things that I wished someone had said to me," said Regina Townsend, a Chicago-area youth-services outreach librarian and writer who began the Broken Brown Egg as a way of addressing what she saw as a troubling silence surrounding the disease of infertility, particularly within the African American community. Her posts can be deeply personal, about her own experience with infertility, the adoption process, and foster care; humorous and chatty, about surviving the baby aisle at Target; or serious and informative, about health or reproductive activism. And, while her journey isn't over yet—she and her husband began the IVF process in 2015—Regina has blogged and written about infertility consistently, on a number of platforms, for six years. "I often want to quit and I get quiet when I'm in that head space," she told me, "but then I shake it off and move forward because I know that someone needs to hear my voice, or just have me say, 'I get it, and I see you, and you're not alone.'"

Creating that missing community is a common motivator for activists—but anger works too. Candace Trinchieri traveled from Los Angeles to D.C. for her first RESOLVE Advocacy Day, a chance to meet with members of Congress about bills affecting reproductive health and family building, in the middle of an IVF cycle—her ninth. "I was pissed off," she remembered. "I wanted to vent at people. But anger is such an easy emotion to have."

For Candace and her husband, their long reproductive journey was complicated by race. Candace is African American, her husband is Italian American, and when they were advised to consider donor eggs, Candace was surprised to find that their options were limited if they wanted the child to resemble both of them. Browsing websites listing hundreds of potential donors, Candace said there were plenty of white and Asian donors but only a handful of African Americans. At her own RESOLVE support group, she tried talking about this frustration, and her eventual determination that she'd settle for a "brown" or multiracial egg donor, but found that the other members, who were mostly white, didn't want to hear her story.

"People of color are usually comfortable talking about race, because we live it every day. But if you're not a person of color, talking about it can make you defensive," she explained. "I felt all of this negativity coming back at me. They wanted to know, 'Why do you care about the color?'"

Candace walked out of that meeting but didn't leave RESOLVE for good. She returned for her first Advocacy Day, in 2013, hoping not only to argue for better laws and protections, but also to draw attention to the need to reach out to diverse communities, which she felt were underrepresented in support groups and RE clinics. "In the waiting room, every face you see is white. Looking at the literature, every face you see is white," she said. "It's extremely isolating."

She went on to become RESOLVE's vice chair of policy for Advocacy Day, drawing on her professional experience in event planning and nonprofit development. She began working to better prepare volunteers new to lobbying. Candace and her husband have raised more than $20,000 through RESOLVE's Southern California Walk of Hope, expanding it from one city to three. With a friend, she is starting a new RESOLVE support group in Los Angeles, open to all but geared to people of color, who she says face an "extra stigma" when dealing with infertility and struggle to find safe or welcoming places to share their experience.

And she became a mother, adopting, with her husband, a baby boy who looks a lot like the genetic child they might have had. Her adoption story is as close to ideal as any infertile couple could imagine—the birth mother chose them at fourteen weeks and allowed Candace to accompany her for ultrasounds and for both Candace and her husband to be present at the birth. "I held her leg while she pushed," Candace remembered. "I got to cut the umbilical cord."

Candace's personal fight made her a better advocate for reproductive equality. "I don't want anyone else to have my struggle," she said. So she travels, speaks publicly about her story, and researches laws affecting infertile couples and individuals. In 2014 and 2015 she worked especially on the Adoption Tax Credit Refundability Act, which would provide tax relief to all adoptive families, not just families with higher incomes, and on the

Women Veterans and Other Health Care Improvements Act, which would extend IVF and other fertility coverage to severely wounded and female veterans. Candace wants people to understand that infertility is not a choice but a destructive, treatable disease affecting not just a few people but many, and from every background. "I go into every Advocacy Day asking people if they know what *one in eight* means," she said, referring to the chance a couple has experienced infertility. "*One in eight* means that it's someone you know, and maybe they're not being treated. It should be a no-brainer that this disease is covered by insurance."

In 2014, Facebook and Apple attracted a wave of criticism not for restricting insurance coverage but expanding it. Both companies announced that they would cover the cost of egg freezing and storage for their employees and covered spouses, allowing women "to do the best work of their lives," according to a press release from Apple. Some claimed that the coverage was coercive, forcing women to choose between motherhood and careers. These critics worried that women might fear choosing their own "natural" time to have a child, at least until they reached a certain career threshold, and argued that both companies would better serve women and families by providing for work-life balance. Medical ethicists cautioned that egg freezing, once classified as experimental and recommended primarily for women about to undergo chemotherapy, is no guarantee that participating women will be able to have a child when they choose—success is dependent on the quality of the eggs at the time of cryopreservation and generally declines with age.

While it's easy to see how corporations benefit if some of their best workers delay childbearing, and while work-life balance is a crucial goal, it feels presumptuous to worry about these women, who are among the most well informed, privileged, and powerful on the planet. But for about two weeks in October, after the news of coverage broke, the story was reported and commented on in every newspaper and magazine I read. DON'T BE FOOLED, ran the headlines. EGG FREEZING BETTER FOR COMPANIES, NOT WOMEN.

Like a number of women who have benefitted from ART, I found the media coverage troubling. First, it seemed to ignore that Plan B family creation is an increasingly common reality and suggested that medicalization degraded the conception experience. Writing for the *New Yorker* website, beneath a photograph of a storage tank filled with test tubes and liquid nitrogen, Rebecca Mead commented that "the inclusion of egg freezing as an employee benefit partakes of the techno-utopian fantasy on which companies like Facebook and Apple subsist— the conviction that there must be a solution to every problem, an answer to every question, a response to every need, if only the right algorithm can be found." Other writers compared the company policies to the coercive dystopian atmosphere of Aldous Huxley's *Brave New World,* in which women submit to egg-harvesting ovariectomies "for the good of Society, not to mention the fact that it carries a bonus amounting to six months' salary." Some articles reported that the two companies were paying women *to* freeze their eggs, rather than offering egg freezing as a covered medical benefit. Most mentioned the dollar amount, *up to $20,000,* reinforcing the discomfort many have associating money and reproduction.

Seven weeks after my daughter's birth, I started a new job as a visiting writer at a university. That position was temporary, but it was followed by a yearlong visitorship at another university and, finally, an offer to stay. It's in many ways a dream job, a chance to work with wonderful colleagues and bright graduate and undergraduate students and to focus far more time on my writing than I could as a K–12 teacher. The position comes with better benefits than I've had in years, including eight weeks of paid maternity leave and an assurance that having a child will provide more time on the tenure clock. That doesn't mean that now, or even a year from now, is the right time to think about adding to my family. I pay quarterly to keep my frozen embryos on ice and sometimes have nightmares that I've missed a payment or that they were accidentally thawed. Maybe Richard and I won't choose to have a second child, but I'm grateful that we don't have to make that decision immediately, that I can focus on my career and family while we figure it out. If our frozen embryos are part of a techno-utopia, I believe it is an empowering one.

I'm lucky, and so are Facebook's and Apple's salaried, noncontract employees, who in addition to egg freezing receive fourteen to twenty-two weeks of paid maternity leave, plus coverage for IVF, adoption, and surrogacy costs. Less fortunate are the women who work almost everywhere else in America, like the women in Ann Bell's study, who in addition to lacking financial or insurance resources have trouble even interesting physicians in their infertility. "Most doctors try to talk you out of getting pregnant," one woman explained.

What is perhaps most problematic, and least surprising, about the interest generated by Apple's and Facebook's announcements is its reinforcement of stereotypes: rich, educated women are the ones most at risk for infertility or childlessness; poor women are hyperfertile, popping out kids in their teens and twenties. All are subject to second-guessing and commentary over what should be a private choice.

And an accessible one. When the Patient Protection and Affordable Care Act was upheld by the Supreme Court in 2012, I got my dad an extra-large black T-shirt that read, in white letters, "Health Reform Still a BFD." The shirt referenced a moment in 2010 when Joe Biden was caught on live microphone, telling the president that the passage of the PPACA was "a big fucking deal." That law *was* a big fucking deal for my family, and for the country, finally putting decent health care within reach for millions of uninsured and underinsured people. For my parents, the PPACA meant that they wouldn't lose coverage after my father's heart surgeries or because they live in a county with no doctors. It meant that hospital bills wouldn't force them into medical bankruptcy.

My mom often borrows the shirt—on her tiny frame, it's a dress—and wears it to Democratic fund-raisers in King and Queen County and sometimes the local pharmacy, where prescriptions cost less than they used to. Sometimes she gets a hard time from Tea Party types grumbling about Obamacare, but, more and more, people are supportive. They're getting used to the idea that health care is a right, not a privilege.

And if health care is a right we should expect, then so is the care of our reproductive health, which is not just absence of disease but the ability to make choices—when or if (and how) you'll have a child or children. I'm with Margaret, with Barbara, with Regina, with Candace. With Mark and Rachel, and Gabe and Todd, and Nate and Parul and Willis.

Waiting is a part of life and can build appreciation and wonder into the life you finally achieve. But you shouldn't have to wait forever.

Epilogue

...

Jamani, the gorilla at the North Carolina Zoo, was a mother only briefly to the baby she carried in 2011. That highly publicized birth ended sadly, with an infant the humans didn't have time to name; something went wrong, and he died. Jamani's keepers closed her exhibit to visitors and allowed her to hold and carry the baby until she made peace with the loss. She did not allow Nkosi and Acacia, the other gorillas in her troop, to get close to the infant but spent the day holding him, cleaning him, and trying to stimulate movement and feeding. Eventually, she set the infant down and moved away.

When I heard about the stillbirth, I thought about something I once unhappily claimed in my support group: it's all just different paths to misery. It was a down time in our group, with every month bringing news of failed IVFs, unexpected surgeries, problems communicating with doctors. I was talking about the risks we all took, through treatment, with our health and finances and happiness, but also about the likelihood that success would never deliver the lives we spent so long fantasizing about. No one corrected me—maybe because they were too kind, or maybe they suspected I might be right.

But that wasn't the end of Jamani's story. Less than a year later, she was pregnant again, along with a new enclosure mate, Olympia, a bossy sixteen-year-old who'd also been cleared for breeding with Nkosi. Ultrasounds indicated healthy pregnancies, with both gorillas due within weeks of each other.

"We held back," said Aaron Jesue, who had by then cared for the zoo's shifting gorilla population for nearly a decade. "We were very excited when Jamani became pregnant the first time, but how do you react if something goes wrong?"

Planning for the gorillas' reproductive future is a significant part of Jesue's job and involves frequent conference calls with other zoos, consultation with the Species Survival Plan, and trips to conferences across the country. In the zoo's mixed-sex group, female gorillas not cleared by the SSP for breeding with Nkosi, their lone silverback, were given birth control. Jamani and Olympia both conceived quickly. Acacia, the oldest female, took the Pill.

On August 4, 2012, Jamani gave birth to a healthy male the keepers named Bomassa; Olympia followed less than a month later with Apollo, another male. A single pregnancy is unusual for captive gorillas at any zoo, but to have two closely spaced, successful births, two healthy infants born within the same group, is almost unheard of. Despite the zoo's low-key announcements, word spread—by Twitter and Facebook, telephone and email—and in late August the keepers had to set up queues to keep hundreds of visitors at a time from overcrowding the two-acre enclosure's small viewing area. Those who couldn't visit in person could browse Apollo and Bomassa's baby books online or comment on their development in short video clips posted to the zoo's Facebook page.

"It was intense," said Jesue, that rare sort of person who does exactly what he dreamed of doing as a child. He felt closest to Nkosi, the zoo's silverback—it was the majestic adult males that inspired him to become a gorilla keeper—but understood why people would wait in a long line, at the end of a hot North Carolina summer, to glimpse the tiny infants clinging to their mothers. "People love the babies. We look at them and see something about ourselves, our families."

I didn't visit the newborns, though I remember thinking— selfishly, nonsensically—that Jamani's success boded well for my own reproductive future and happiness. I had followed and written about her first pregnancy and loss, and now, just a year later, I browsed her baby book online. One photo appealed to me especially—a close-up of Jamani resting her great chin protectively on Bomassa's head. His large eyes shine within his tiny, heart-shaped face; Jamani gazes upward with a look of reverie, as if she finds everything about him—his infant smell, his soft fur, the weight of his body—intoxicating. I opened other web pages and plugged my own relevant numbers (age, number of years trying, past failures) into databases that calculated IVF success rates. Sometimes 27 percent, sometimes 24 percent, depending on the database. Perhaps one day this would all be a memory for me too.

What the visitors to the North Carolina Zoo probably missed, and what the newspapers didn't report, is something that happened just a few days after the second gorilla was born, when no one, not even a keeper, was watching. Olympia, newly postpartum and socially dominant, kidnapped Jamani's three-week-old son, Bomassa, one night and began caring for him—nursing him, holding him chest-to-chest, and keeping him away from danger—alongside her own newborn. Physically larger than Olympia but ranked last in the three-female hierarchy, Jamani made cries of distress, spun in circles, and ran from one edge of the enclosure to the other. The keepers, who'd seen Jamani cradling her stillborn baby just a year earlier, waited in anguish to see if she'd take Bomassa back, but all she managed was some halfhearted charging and huffing in Olympia's direction.

Infant kidnapping is not uncommon among primates, who

take babies for a number of reasons: as a form of infanticide, clearing the way for their own genetic success; to increase their social status; to gain experience with caregiving; and sometimes because they are just very interested in babies. Olympia had a healthy infant who was not threatened by the birth of Bomassa, and she was on top, socially. Why would she add to her workload—so considerable that gorillas typically space births at least four years apart—by adopting a second baby?

Through phone calls with zoos where Olympia and Jamani spent their early years, Jesue and his colleagues determined that both gorillas were influenced by the maternal behavior they saw when they were young. Olympia lived at Zoo Atlanta with a mother of twins and must have thought that two babies were ideal. In San Diego, where Jamani was raised, infant sharing was common and tolerated. They both expressed patterns of behavior they'd already seen, images lodged not in their genetic code but in the captivity-limited memories they had of motherhood and family life. *This is how an adult gorilla behaves,* we can imagine Olympia thinking as she loped around the enclosure, two infants clinging to her chest. *Surely she'll give him back,* we can picture Jamani deciding, as her mammaries swelled painfully with milk for Bomassa. *That's what mother gorillas do.*

It took five days of watching and waiting for the gorilla keepers to decide that enough was enough; they finally sedated Olympia and gave Bomassa back to Jamani. She was able to nurse him because the keepers had painstakingly pumped her milk using a human breast pump in the days when she and Bomassa were separated (submission to pumping is part of their maternal training), and she responded to the return of her infant almost as if nothing had ever happened.

"She's a great mother," Jesue told me, praising Jamani's patience with her son, her gentle discipline. We were standing by the enclosure's viewing area while Bomassa and Apollo, by then two years old, wrestled and chased each other through the tall grass. "Olympia is a great mother too," he added, though he acknowledged that she was also fairly permissive.

So much had happened since Apollo's and Bomassa's births that Jesue admitted feeling stunned when he thought about this group's reproductive history. "It's been a roller coaster," he said. In 2012 a third female, Acacia, was cleared for breeding with Nkosi; like Jamani and Olympia, she conceived quickly. But, unlike with those two, Acacia's birth was difficult, more than twenty-four hours long, and the keepers and zoo veterinarians decided to give her an emergency cesarean. Though the surgery went well and the infant was healthy—"He was the prettiest, strongest one," another keeper told me—he died suddenly after being returned to her, and the keepers, for the second time in two years, stood by helplessly while a new mother came to terms with her loss. Later that year, Nkosi died suddenly of encephalitis.

Jesue had a hard time thinking about the loss of Nkosi, affectionately called Nik by the keepers. He'd been a patient, gentle father, participating in infant care beyond expectations for gorilla fathers.

I asked him what would happen to Acacia, who was also, by all accounts, a good caretaker, frequently playing with Bomassa and Apollo but staying clear, for the most part, of the infant-snatching, socially dominant Olympia. The keepers expected to welcome another silverback to the group, a role model for the two young males. Would Acacia conceive again?

No, Jesue told me. It was too dangerous. They planned to move Acacia to another zoo—her third—and hoped that she could serve as an allomother, or motherly caregiver, or even a surrogate in case another gorilla rejected her infant. *That happens more often than you'd think,* he said, before leaving to help with the lunchtime feeding.

I stayed behind and watched, paying particular attention to Acacia, who was lounging in a pile of hay near the glass, eating the rich seeds, but who also appeared to keep one eye on the dominant, reproductively successful Olympia, foraging for the last of the celery and lettuce tossed down at feeding time.

Small crowds—schoolchildren, families—pressed close to the viewing area. Without Jesue to correct them, a few visitors confused Jamani, hulking on the far side of the enclosure while Bomassa scampered about, for Nkosi. "There's the dad. See him?"

"They're just like you," more than one adult said to a child of four or five. "Always into something."

Crowds gathered, moved on, then gathered again.

"I bet the gorillas think they're just like us," a girl of seven or eight offered. "They don't even know they're called gorillas."

It's easy, tempting, to project our own stories onto more public ones. We see our struggles and experiences and personalities mirrored in gorillas at the zoo, in characters in films and books. I look at Acacia and see traces of my infertile self, a lurking outsider who would have made a good mother, if only. Or I rewatch *Raising Arizona* and notice the way everyone is softened by the presence of the smiling, cooing baby. The prison escapees who kidnap Nathan Junior (again!) for the ransom money also steal toys to amuse him with; the materialistic and temperamental Nathan Arizona, relieved to have his boy returned, forgives both Hi and Ed. We're warned against these temptations to project—nothing in our own complex lives is so simple as an anthropomorphized gorilla or a Hollywood caper.

Gorillas don't know what we call them, it's true; watching Acacia and Jamani and Olympia, I have the sense that they hardly regard us at all. They focus instead on immediate, gorilla things: *Where will the last of the lettuce get tossed? How far can I afford to let my infant roam while I look for the lettuce?* They live in the moment, unconcerned with the passing of time, with what's missing. We can't know their minds, but they seem content.

And yet there is something beautiful about the human mind, its ability to travel into the past or the future by force of will. At the end of *Raising Arizona,* Hi and Ed confess to Nathan Arizona that they plan to split up—they're both too selfish and unrealistic, they've realized, to make it as a couple. The gruff Nathan tells them to sleep on it, "at least one night," and the movie ends with an image of Hi's bandaged, sleeping face and scenes from his dream. He describes his dream self as "a floating spirit, visiting things to come," and sees the young Nathan Junior opening the Christmas present of a football, sent to him by "a kindly couple who preferred to remain unknown" and, later, scoring a winning touchdown in a college game. Then Hi sees an even more distant future, years and years away: an old couple visited by smiling children and grandchildren, the whole family sitting down in a wood-paneled dining room to a table of food that appears endless in its bounty.

"Was it wishful thinking? Was I just fleein' reality, like I know I'm liable to do?" Hi asks. "It seemed real. It seemed like us. And it seemed like well . . . our home." We don't glimpse the faces of the older couple, but we see what they see: the handsome adult children, the grandchildren with Sunday clothes and party manners. The banner that reads WELCOME HOME KIDS.

Imagining the future is not only a way of fleeing reality but of courting it. It's a balm and a gift, as well as the force behind all the things we want that happen not by lucky accident but by effort: the better job, the published story or book, the comfortable retirement, the family of two or three or four. "You gotta just keep tryin'," Nathan Arizona told Hi and Ed, "and hope medical science catches up with you." If it didn't work, he added, they still had each other.

Keep trying. Be content. How do you reconcile those two messages? How do you do both at once? I turned those questions over for a long time: not quite content, not actively trying, while all around me other people tried harder. Nate and Parul, with their long journey to their son. Margaret with her medical odyssey. Candace and Regina with their activism and message of inclusion. Dr. Ramos with her determination to innovate on behalf of hopeful patients.

By the time I was pregnant, a new cicada cohort was due to emerge: the seventeen-year cicadas, predicted to be even more numerous and raucous than the thirteen-year group whose constant hum accompanied my first rounds of ART failure. Reports suggested that these cicadas, Brood II, might outnumber humans in their range six hundred to one.

Instead the 2013 emergence was a bust, at least where I live—no undulating song, no exoskeletal forest carpet. In May, when we expected them, I'd passed my worried first trimester and was regularly hiking through the woods and along the river. I listened for the cicadas and let my mind wander. To the past: not to the last major emergence, when the cicadas' abundance was overwhelming, but to a long-ago Virginia brood that emerged when I was in elementary school. For about a month their husks littered every path to the lake where my brother and I spent most afternoons. We collected them delicately and attached their ghostly bodies to our clothes until we were covered, like the tree trunks surrounding the lake. It was our mother who first showed us how to gather cicadas without crushing them.

And, like Hi, I thought about the future. I could imagine one day—maybe in nine years, when the thirteen-year cicadas return—reliving the experience with my own child. But imagination has its limits—there was a flat quality to what I saw, an absence of sound. A distance between the imagining self and the imagined one.

For me, having and raising a child, who happened to be conceived through IVF, has been more magical than my mind was able to conjure.

I'm glad I didn't know before I had her. I don't think I could have borne it.

In the months after our daughter was born, emboldened by our risk taking, Richard and I began an addition to our one-bedroom house. I often met our contractors in the driveway with Beatrice wrapped in one of the slings that creates the warm, chest-to-chest closeness gorillas have, and, though the contractors could see only the top of her head, they solicitously offered praise: she was so beautiful, so sweet.

"Imagine if there was only one baby in the whole world," began Mr. Cheek, the mason we hired to build our foundation. He pointed at Beatrice, sleeping against my chest, as if she were the imagined only baby. "Wherever that baby was, we'd put down our things and go see it. If that baby was in California, we'd all go to California."

Mr. Cheek, a father and grandfather, knew nothing of our long wait for Beatrice; that was not his point. He knew something bigger, more profound: each baby is born not just to her parents, but to the world surrounding her. To neighbors, friends, teachers, enclosure mates. To ex-cons and allomothers and cousins and grandmothers, who will each want a peek and will each have some impact.

In my sleep-deprived haze, I pictured myself, Richard, and Bea in a kind of enclosure on a cliff above the Pacific, with a queue of curious well-wishers snaking all the way to the desert. Given how long it took us to have her, the many people involved in the process, the image felt strangely fitting. I now have a number of friends who have had babies through some form of medical intervention, through intrauterine insemination and IVF and medicated cycles, with the help of donor eggs or embryos, pills or injectable drugs. It's common for people in our circle to call our children miracles, to see our experiences as singular and exclusive, to think about how close we came to not having them. But this is true of every baby, every romantic pairing, every relationship on earth—we are all terrifyingly beholden to risk and fear and luck, to longings that arrive as expected or, for some of us, emerge from some deep, surprising well we didn't know we had.

Mr. Cheek repeated himself, as if to test my agreement.

"You're probably right," I told him. "I'd go."

ACKNOWLEDGMENTS

I'm very grateful to the journals that first published these essays, sometimes in different forms: "The Art of Waiting" and "Baby Fever" appeared in *Orion* ("The Art of Waiting" was reprinted in *Harper's* and the 2013 William Hazlitt Prize edition); "Imaginary Children" appeared in *Ecotone;* "Visible Life" appeared in *Slate;* and "The Whole House" appeared in the *Sun.*

Thanks to Katie Dublinski, my editor, for her vast patience and wisdom; to Maria Massie, my agent, for her encouragement and assistance; to Michael Taeckens, my publicist, for his talent and dedication; and to all of the wonderful people at Graywolf, especially Fiona McCrae, Marisa Atkinson, Erin Kottke, and Caroline Nitz. I feel so lucky to have my books published alongside Graywolf's other titles.

Thank you to the North Carolina Arts Council and the National Endowment for the Arts for financial support while I worked on this book, and to the Durham Arts Council for support during my book tour. Thank you, also, to the institutions that gave me a home as I wrote—a temporary one at Lenoir-Rhyne University, where I was a visitor, and a more lasting one at North Carolina State University, where I teach now. I'm grateful to my many inspiring students and my brilliant colleagues, especially Rand Brandes at Lenoir-Rhyne, and Wilton Barnhardt, Jill McCorkle, John Kessel, Cat Warren, and Dorianne Laux at NCSU.

Thank you to my friends and fellow writers who helped and encouraged me with the manuscript: Meaghan Mulholland, Jon

Mozes, Krista Bremer, Duncan Murrell, Dan Kois, Andrew Park, Jonathan Farmer, Catey Christiansen, Emily L. Smith, Anna Lena Phillips, Hannah Fries, Andrew Blechman, Michelle Latiolais, Margaret Zamos-Monteith, Sophie Shaw, Courtney Fitzpatrick, John Railey, David Potorti, and Banu Valladares. Thank you also to the caregivers who made it possible for me to teach and write after Bea was born, especially Buttons Boggs, Laura Denning, Sophie Shaw, Kaela Self, and Sylvia Grant.

And to the many people who agreed to be interviewed for this book: I am so grateful for your generosity, thoughtfulness, poise, and insight. Thank you to the scientists, doctors, and researchers who patiently answered questions and reviewed drafts, in particular Leslie Digby, Anna Rotkirch, Aaron Jesue, Marni Rosner, Stephen Young, and Silvia Ramos. Thank you to Dr. Young and Dr. Ramos for helping me not only with my book but with my life. And to RESOLVE, a vital source of support, information, and lasting friendships.

Thank you to my family for allowing me to represent parts of our life here—my endlessly supportive parents, Buttons and Terry Boggs, in particular.

And to Richard Allen: you are always my first and best reader. Thank you for the endless draft reads, discussions, and research help—this book would not exist without you.

And to Beatrice: the best person I know.

SELECTED RESOURCES

A collection of the resources I mention in the book or that were suggested to me by people I interviewed follows. If you have additional suggestions you'd like to contribute, please visit my website, belleboggs .com, where I'm gathering a longer list.

SUPPORT GROUPS

RESOLVE: The National Infertility Association (resolve.org): A national nonprofit that provides education and resources for, and advocates on behalf of, women and men experiencing infertility or reproductive disorders. Their website offers medical information about infertility; suggestions for emotional coping; practical guides for interviewing doctors, adoption professionals, and therapists; guides to family-building options including adoption and ART; and links to online support communities. RESOLVE also offers free training to people who want to start peer-led support groups, and resolve.org offers contact information for its 261 support groups in forty-four states, plus D.C. The support group I mention throughout the book is a general RESOLVE infertility support group. Some cities offer more specific groups that are focused, for example, on secondary infertility or adoption.

Share Pregnancy and Infant Loss Support (nationalshare.org): "A community for anyone who experiences the tragic death of a baby." Share's seventy-five chapters in twenty-nine states welcome parents, grandparents, siblings, and other family members to their support groups and events, and their website provides information for bereaved family members and their caregivers.

Fertility for Colored Girls (fertilityforcoloredgirls.org): A nonprofit devoted to education and awareness about reproductive health in the African American community. The organization has chapters in Chicago, D.C., Richmond, and Atlanta and also hosts online events and fund-raisers.

ONLINE COMMUNITIES AND BLOGS

The Broken Brown Egg (thebrokenbrownegg.org): Regina Townsend's blog about her own experience with infertility, including discussions and education about infertility in the African American community, as well as a list of African American and minority infertility resources that Townsend has collected.

Inspire (inspire.com): A privately held company that offers online patient communities for people with a number of health and wellness concerns, including infertility. They are partnered with RESOLVE in two online communities, one focused on finding a resolution for infertility, and the other on living after infertility resolution. More at inspire.com/partners/resolve/.

ADOPTION INFORMATION

The Noah Z. M. Goetz Foundation (nzmgfoundation.org): Offers education and financial assistance to infertile couples and individuals pursuing domestic adoption. Domestic Adoption 101 is a two-hour group workshop offered in the Triangle area of North Carolina for a small fee; Domestic Adoption 102 is offered one-on-one and is available in person or by phone or videoconference. The nonprofit foundation also offers grants of $1,000 each, which are intended to help offset the cost of infant domestic adoption.

Adoptive Families **magazine** (adoptivefamilies.com): A quarterly digital magazine for adoptive-parents-to-be and families raising children through adoption. Their website provides access to articles about every stage of the adoption process.

Adoption.net: An online resource for parents, birth mothers, and adoptees that provides information and online forums about foster care and adoption.

Creating a Family (creatingafamily.org): A national nonprofit organization providing information and resources about infertility and pre- and post-adoptive families. Creating a Family hosts a weekly radio show that is available online, publishes a newsletter, and is active on Facebook, Twitter, and Pinterest.

CHILD-FREE LIVING

Infertility and the Creative Spirit, **cowritten by clinical psychologist Roxane Head Dinkin and history professor Robert J. Dinkin**: The authors, who could not have children themselves, use the life stories of seven prominent women to make the argument that those who want children but cannot have them often channel their desire into lasting creative accomplishments.

Silent Sorority: A (Barren) Woman Gets Busy, Angry, Lost and Found by **Pamela Mahoney Tsigdinos:** A memoir of Tsigdinos's experience of moving on after unsuccessful fertility treatments. Tsigdinos also maintains a blog with insights and commentary about living child-free after infertility on her website, silentsorority.com.

RESOLVE also offers resources and personal stories related to child-free living at www.resolve.org/family-building-options/living_childfree/.

GRANTS AND FINANCIAL ASSISTANCE

Pay It Forward Fertility Foundation (payitforwardfertility.org): A nonprofit organization providing financial assistance to couples who could not otherwise afford IVF.

The Tinina Q. Cade Foundation (cadefoundation.org): A nonprofit that provides information and financial assistance to needy couples embarking on medical fertility treatment or adoption. The foundation's website has a lengthy list of additional resources related to grants for adoption and fertility treatment, access to discount medications, and fund-raising.

See the **Noah Z. M. Goetz Foundation**, above.

THERAPY AND MENTAL HEALTH

"Recovery from Traumatic Loss: A Study of Women Living without Children after Infertility" by Marni Rosner (repository.upenn.edu/cgi /viewcontent.cgi?article=1020&context=edissertations_sp2): A comprehensive guide to the common struggles of infertile women. Dr. Rosner is also a psychotherapist practicing in New York and treats individuals and couples struggling with anxiety, relationship issues, trauma, loss, and infertility.

Open Path Psychotherapy Collective (openpathcollective.org): A nationwide group of licensed mental-health professionals who have agreed to provide in-office psychotherapeutic treatment for rates that range between thirty and fifty dollars a session. The website is searchable by specialty, including infertility, and some therapists offer remote therapy through Skype.

Path2Parenthood (path2parenthood.org): A nonprofit "committed to helping people create their families of choice." Their website has a searchable database of mental-health professionals specializing in infertility and family building.

FOR ART PATIENTS

The Centers for Disease Control and Prevention (cdc.gov/ART/index .html): A federal agency that collects and publishes information related to ART and fertility. The CDC releases an annual report of statistics and success rates from more than 440 ART clinics nationwide, and their page of patient resources includes links to clinical trials.

The Society for Assisted Reproductive Technology (sart.org): A nonprofit that collects and publishes information from more than 90 percent of the ART clinics in America. Their website allows you to search for clinics by zip code or state and view corresponding IVF success rates by age, diagnosis, treatment type, and number of embryos transferred.

The American Society for Reproductive Medicine (reproductivefacts .org): A nonprofit that offers patient information and outreach. Their website includes access to studies and medical journals, fact sheets and information booklets (also in Spanish), information about fertility after cancer treatment, a state-by-state guide to insurance laws, and educational videos.

LEGAL ISSUES

Love's Promises **by Martha Ertman:** A book about the power of contracts in what Ertman calls "Plan B" family formation. Ertman provides a detailed overview of the way formal and informal contracts affect families, including those formed through assisted reproductive technologies and surrogacy. The book also includes sample contracts for cohabitation, coparenting, and third-party reproduction.

The Family Equality Council (familyequality.org): An organization that "connects, supports, and represents the three million parents who are lesbian, gay, bisexual, transgender and queer in this country and their six million children." Their website is a good resource for information about protecting the legal status and rights of family members and children, as well as state-by-state guides to nondiscrimination laws, adoption and foster-care laws, parental-recognition laws, and family-leave laws.

ADVOCACY

Center for Infertility Justice (resolve.org/get-involved/the-center-for-infertility-justice/federal-legislation/): This RESOLVE program monitors state and federal legislative issues related to infertility, the practice of ART, and adoption, including the Family Act, the Adoption Tax Credit Refundability Act, Reproductive Treatment for Certain Disabled Veterans, and the Women Veterans and Families Health Services Act. The program also lobbies state and federal legislatures to pass laws that favor the interests of infertile people.

EUGENICS PROGRAMS AND THE FIGHT FOR COMPENSATION IN AMERICA

Rage to Redemption in the Sterilization Age **by John Railey:** A powerful overview of the history of the eugenics-based sterilization program in North Carolina and the ultimately successful fight for compensation for its victims. Railey, a longtime reporter, columnist, and editor for the *Winston-Salem Journal,* has written about eugenics-based sterilization for more than a decade.

My piece of long-form journalism about eugenics-based sterilization and North Carolina's victims and advocates, *"For the Public Good,"* was published in 2013 by the *New New South.*

NOTES

Some of the people I interviewed chose to be quoted pseudonymously. I have indicated the use of pseudonyms in the notes.

5 **My name is called, and a doctor I've never met:** Fifteen to eighteen percent is the chance per cycle my doctor estimated for me early in my IUI treatment, but it's unlikely—or at least unclear—that my chances were ever this high, given the combination of factors that contributed to our infertility.

Over the course of my infertility treatment, I tried three different protocols: letrozole (brand name Femara), an aromatase inhibitor that's prescribed off label to stimulate ovarian response; letrozole plus intrauterine insemination; and finally IVF. Though each treatment had the same goal, it was interesting to me how much more attentive my care was as the cost increased. For example, I took letrozole for eight months (it was prescribed by my gynecologist) and never had an ultrasound to monitor its effectiveness (even after my dosage was increased when I did not become pregnant). When I began IUI treatment in a reproductive endocrinology clinic, we discovered via ultrasound that the prescribed dosage was producing four to five mature follicles per cycle, which is potentially dangerous (my IUI cycle was canceled to prevent the risk of multiples). During my IUI cycles, ovulation was predicted by an over-the-counter ovulation predictor kit, but IVF involved a team of clinicians and a schedule of blood draws, phone calls, and ultrasounds.

5 **Humans have a long history of imposing various forms of birth control and reproductive technologies on animals:** More recently, when the northern white rhinoceros population dwindled to five because of poaching and habitat loss, scientists considered IVF a possible means of staving off the species' extinction. Only

one female rhino, a thirty-one-year-old resident of a Czech zoo plagued with uterine cysts, was of reproductive age. She died of a ruptured cyst in July 2015; scientists collected her healthy ovary in the hopes of eventually maturing the eggs and making use of her genetic material. If they are able to use IVF successfully, the resulting embryo will likely be gestated in a closely related subspecies.

20 **The first evolutionary psychologist:** I was introduced to the long-standing debate over the so-called childbearing instinct (versus the sex drive) through the fascinating work of Anna Rotkirch, a family sociologist whose study "All That She Wants Is A(nother) Baby?," was the first description I found of the biological sources of child-longing. Rotkirch's "What Is 'Baby Fever'?," published in *The New Evolutionary Social Science: Human Nature, Social Behavior, and Social Change* (edited by Heinz-Jürgen Niedenzu, Tamás Meleghy, and Peter Meyer), informs this chapter as well, especially the discussion of the function of baby fever for those facing barriers such as infertility or the absence of a relationship. Rotkirch also generously emailed with me about her work.

21 **In America, 62 percent of reproductive-age women use some form of birth control; at current rates, 30 percent of American women will have had abortions by their forty-fifth birthdays:** These statistics come from studies completed in the past ten years. I found the birth control statistic in "Current Contraceptive Use in the United States, 2006–2010, and Changes in Patterns of Use Since 1995," by J. Jones, W. D. Mosher, and K. Daniels, published in *National Health Statistics Reports,* no. 60 (2012). The abortion statistic comes from "Changes in Abortion Rates between 2000 and 2008 and Lifetime Incidence of Abortion," a paper by R. K. Jones and M. L. Kavanaugh, published in *Obstetrics and Gynecology* 117, no. 6 (2011).

25 **"an emotion which may be typical for societies where women have many choices":** This quote comes from Rotkirch's "What Is 'Baby Fever'?," which provides an overview of her baby-fever research.

30 **Aside from possibly imparting a genetic proceptive tendency:** I'm using *proceptive* as Rotkirch defines it: "behavior that favors

childbearing and is the opposite of contraception." She cites a 1999 study published in *Population and Development Review* by Hans-Peter Kohler, Joseph L. Rodgers, and Kaare Christensen ("Is Fertility Behavior in Our Genes? Findings from a Danish Twin Study"), which examined the first attempted pregnancy among Danish twins born from 1870 to 1910 (a high-fertility period) and from 1953 to 1964 (a time of lower fertility). The female twins in the first group showed little genetic influence in their proceptive behavior, but among the latter group, this influence increased. So baby fever may be something we inherit from our mothers and grandmothers, more argument that the desire for children is in-born. This term has also been used by Warren B. Miller, a U.S. demographer.

30 **Pronatalism is the idea that parenting is a normalizing rite of passage:** My understanding of the impact of pronatalism on infertile women is influenced by reading Marni Rosner's dissertation, "Recovery from Traumatic Loss: A Study of Women Living without Children after Infertility" (2012). The details about the history of pronatalism in America come from Elaine Tyler May's *Barren in the Promised Land: Childless Americans and the Pursuit of Happiness* (Harvard University Press, 1995).

45 **I am not Catholic, or even religious, but I notice that my state-provided health insurance coverage for infertility matches the recommendations in the *Donum Vitae:*** The health insurance plan I had at the time of my IUI and IVF treatment was BlueCross BlueShield of North Carolina's health plan for teachers and state employees. Though my plan covered diagnostic tests and even expensive (and sometimes less effective) procedures to treat structural causes of infertility, such as a blocked fallopian tube, it specifically excluded "artificial means of conception." This re-minded me of the Catholic teaching I'd read regarding IVF, which puzzled me—my insurance was not provided by a religious orga-nization (cross aside). If IVF was less expensive and more effec-tive at overcoming infertility than certain surgeries (for both men and women), why wasn't it covered? Additionally, I wondered why IVF, which can treat both male and female infertility factors, was generally billed to the woman's insurance. If the woman is seen as the patient (because it is her body that receives the treatment of

IVF or IUI), does that make exclusion of coverage discriminatory? In 2012, I spoke by phone about these questions with Barbara Collura, president and CEO of RESOLVE, who has worked for more than a decade on expanding state mandates for infertility coverage. Collura suggested that proponents of more inclusive insurance coverage for infertility face two primary obstacles: lack of medical understanding by some insurance companies, and fundraising deficits among infertility organizations such as RESOLVE. At the time of our interview, Collura lamented that RESOLVE had a budget of $1.2 million a year, or about twenty cents to spend on each of the 7.3 million Americans who struggle with the disease.

47   **Initially, some playgoers and critics struggled:** My descriptions of critical reactions to Albee's play, his correspondence with Leonard Woolf, and his unhappy childhood mostly come from Mel Gussow's excellent *Edward Albee: A Singular Journey*.

69   Miss Anne and Miss Dierdre, the two neighbors from "In the Peanut Hospital," are described pseudonymously.

79   **Until about a hundred years ago, when doctors and scientists began collecting and displaying fetal specimens:** I learned about early concepts of embryos and fetuses from Lynn M. Morgan's *Icons of Life: A Cultural History of Human Embryos*. Morgan's book also guided some of my thinking about the political, social, and emotional challenges of conceptualizing embryonic life.

81   In "Just Adopt," Kate, the name of the birth mother, is a pseudonym. The Alexander family is quoted and described pseudonymously.

88   **Primate mothers have even been documented as oblivious or insensitive to an accidental switch:** Descriptions of primate babies' dependency and the occasional accidental trading of babies (such as an observed example in Brazil, when two experienced muriqui monkeys traded babies by accident, then raised them successfully to adulthood) came from Sarah Hrdy's *Mothers and Others: The Evolutionary Origins of Mutual Understanding*.

95   **But more positively, perhaps the extra embryos created in a cycle can be adopted:** Though the American Society for Reproductive Medicine prefers the term *donation* and an anonymous, nondiscriminatory process, some genetic and intended parents

prefer the screening process and implications of adoption, which can include everything from a home study to the requirement that the intended parents be married heterosexual couples. Nightlight Christian Adoptions (nightlight.org), which began offering cryo-preserved embryos to infertile couples in 1997, describes on its website a mission that suggests embryonic personhood: "Just as each snowflake is frozen, unique and a gift from heaven, so are each of our Snowflake Babies. We hope to help each donated embryo grow, develop and live a full life." Nightlight even offers "waiting embryos" with identified risk factors, including health issues discovered in the genetic family or an assigned lower grade from an embryologist.

101 **North Carolina was one of thirty-three states to pass eugenics legislation:** The *Winston-Salem Journal*'s five-part series "Against Their Will" provides an excellent background on North Carolina's eugenics-based sterilization program, and the paper has had ongoing coverage of issues around compensation. John Railey, who wrote many of the pieces in "Against Their Will" and is an editor at the *Winston-Salem Journal*, published *Rage to Redemption in the Sterilization Age* in 2014. His book looks particularly at the state's coercive actions in sterilizing Nial Cox Ramirez, who was one of the first victims to bring a civil case against the state.

102 *It was a long time ago,* **some legislators claimed:** "You just can't rewrite history. It was a sorry time in this country," then–state senator Don East told the Associated Press in a 2012 interview. "I'm so sorry it happened, but throwing money don't change it, don't make it go away. It still happened."

102 **there is evidence that infertility, as a stressor, is equivalent to the experience of living with cancer, HIV, or other chronic illnesses:** The information about infertility as traumatic loss comes both from Rosner's study and from phone and email interviews with Rosner.

119 **The specialty mail-order pharmacy that miraculously accepted my insurance:** Medication for IVF treatment was not covered under my insurance plan, but somehow the medications prescribed by my doctor were partially paid by insurance, and I paid significantly less than I had been told by the online pharmacy

to expect. Another friend, going through IVF at the same time, under the same insurance plan, was not so lucky. I assumed the unexpected coverage was a clerical error that would be discovered at any time and was so afraid of the error's discovery that I didn't press the issue of another medication, Crinone, which should have been covered after my confirmed pregnancy.

The cost of medication is an unpredictable factor in IVF treatment—you don't know, until your cycle is under way, how much injectable gonadotropin you'll need to stimulate ovarian response. Medication is generally not covered by "cost-share" plans such as the one we purchased and can be approved or denied for coverage by insurance companies based on the treatment protocol (for example, the same injectable drugs might be covered for timed intercourse but not for IVF).

It's also common to have drugs left over, and patients frequently give away or sell this medication at a reduced cost. In my cycle, I received Follistim left over from a friend's completed cycle, just in case I needed it, and when my cycle was done, I passed along my leftover Follistim (and my friend's) to another friend. Doctors and medical organizations warn patients not to accept leftover medication—you don't know if it has been stored properly, for example, especially if you're purchasing it from a stranger. But, with medication sharing one of the only ways patients have to reduce the cost of their cycles, it seems unlikely that the practice will end.

129 **I found reports online:** The information I found regarding Lupron's self-reported adverse events was collected on lupronvictimshub .com, which reported numbers collected from a Freedom of Information Act request to the FDA, and from an article titled "Lupron: Do the Risks Outweigh the Benefits?" on lawyersandsettlements .com. Anyone can make a report of an adverse event or reaction to a prescription or over-the-counter drug using MedWatch, the FDA's online voluntary reporting system. More alarming than any of these reports I found online was a line from Andrew Solomon's *Far from the Tree,* which described Lupron (which is also used as an experimental treatment of severe autism) as "a castration drug that changes the body as profoundly as any medication can."

129 **It would have been possible to limit my exposure:** We talked over a number of treatment protocols with our doctor, who was always patient with our need to compare. Although some studies

("Efficacy and Safety of Ganirelix Acetate versus Leuprolide Acetate in Women undergoing Controlled Ovarian Hyperstimulation," *Fertility and Sterility* 75, no. 1 [2001]) suggest that the antagonist protocol has outcomes almost equal to Lupron down-regulation, the latter has been used for longer.

146 **Dr. Young had a formula: if three times as many embryos as we wished to transfer (for us, that meant three competent embryos) were developing normally on day three, we could wait:** Steven Young later told me, "Interestingly, our new lab is so much better at making blastocysts that we only need two times the number on day three. We are doing a lot more single embryo transfers because of this—about three-fourths of women under thirty-five and probably half of women thirty-five to thirty-seven." Though this data had not been made public yet by SART, he reported that the 2013–2014 pregnancy rate for patients under thirty-five using single embryo transfer was 79 percent.

153 In "Birth Stories," Todd Jensen and Gabe Faibish are pseudonyms.

156 **His organization funded and published a study:** I first learned about this study through NeJaime's article in the *Yale Law Journal*. "My Daddy's Name Is Donor" is a study of 485 adults conceived through sperm donation, and reports fifteen findings, including a sense of confusion and loss among donor-conceived children, higher rates of delinquency and substance abuse among the donor-conceived, and higher rates of divorce in their families.

Before reading this study, I was familiar with some of the arguments about the rights of donor-conceived people through Alana Newman's Anonymous Us project, an online collection of personal stories from people conceived through third-party reproduction. Many of the anonymous narratives on this site express anger at their genetic parents (particularly the donors) and discomfort with the idea that money was exchanged as part of their conception. The searchable database of stories (anonymousus.org) also includes posts from parents who have used or considered third-party reproduction.

The Institute for American Values, which published "My Daddy's Name Is Donor," and many of the participants in Anonymous Us argue against anonymity in gamete donation, which is legal in the United States but prohibited in Britain, Sweden, Norway, the

Netherlands, and Switzerland. The *New York Times* published a discussion of donor anonymity and the question of regulation in their Room for Debate series on September 13, 2011. I was most compelled by two of the editorials. Robert G. Brzyski, chairman of the American Society for Reproductive Medicine's ethics committee, argued that donor gametes and embryos are already subject to genetic and medical screening and that additional requirements could make the donation process even more expensive, and limit access. Sujatha Jesudason, the executive director of Generations Ahead, an advocacy group that focuses on the social justice implications of genetic technologies, expressed concern that additional regulation of ART could set a precedent for additional abortion restrictions, as well as a fear that regulation would disenfranchise more vulnerable populations. "Regulating assisted reproduction could mean higher prices and less economic access for some or could be a political opportunity to legislate morality and deny access to gays and lesbians," she wrote. "This doesn't mean that we don't regulate, but we should be very careful in assessing the costs and benefits of who would be the most affected by restrictions on the fertility industry, and by extension in abortion services."

170 **Couples strained by years of infertility can choose new treatment options:** The first report of preimplantation genetic screening that resulted in a healthy pregnancy was published in 1990. The screening, which is most often undertaken by patients with a poor prognosis or a history of miscarriages or failed IVF treatment, remains controversial and is often what people refer to when they discuss "designer babies," in part because the process can also be used to select for sex. Likewise, many responded in alarm to the news, in 2015, that the UK would become the first country to allow IVF that replaces disease-carrying maternal mitochondria with mitochondria from a donor egg.

171 **But even the definition of *biological* has changed:** "It is clear that genes are not puppeteers directing behavior," writes the anthropologist Sarah Hrdy in *Mother Nature,* her book on biology and the maternal instinct. "A range of non-genetic factors, such as mother's physical condition or social status, the season when she conceived, her own diet or the one she provided her baby, the presence or absence of father—all contribute to individualization."

For this reason Hrdy takes issue with the common misuse of the phrase "biological mother" to refer to the genetic or gestational mother, and the binary thinking behind "nature versus nurture." Further, the evolving field of epigenetics has demonstrated a multitude of ways in which environmental changes (to diet or temperature, for example), can affect the expression of genes, turning them on or off.

184 **These treatments are so much less effective than IVF that most clinics don't even keep careful track of them:** The Fertility Clinic Success Rate and Certification Act of 1992 requires all clinics to report IVF statistics and success rates to the Centers for Disease Control and Prevention. This mandated reporting influences record keeping, Steven Young suggested.

185 **Reading about the mandatory coverage requirements of the fourteen other states:** RESOLVE publishes a useful guide to the insurance coverage mandated in fifteen states (resolve.org/family-building-options/insurance_coverage/state-coverage.html).

193 **But it is also true that infertility is an emotionally punishing experience:** In 1998, the Supreme Court found in *Bragdon v. Abbott* that reproduction is "a major life activity," qualifying infertile people for some protection. Under the Americans with Disabilities Act, forbidding an infertile person from taking time off to pursue fertility treatment may constitute disability discrimination. The exclusion of fertility treatments such as IVF from employer-provided health care is not considered discriminatory under the ADA, because the exclusion applies to everyone, not just the infertile patients. Advocates for the infertile counter that by choosing to exclude from coverage a particular kind of health care, which would be used only by workers experiencing a particular health condition, employers discriminate.

205 **Both companies announced that they would cover the cost of egg freezing and storage:** This coverage was not extended to contract workers, such as receptionists and security, food-service, and maintenance workers.

205 **While it's easy to see how corporations might benefit if some of their best workers delay childbearing, and while work-life balance is a crucial goal, it feels presumptuous to worry about**

these women: Apple, Facebook, and many other tech companies are rightly criticized for vast gender and diversity gaps. In 2015, 69 percent of Apple's workers were male, and, according to an Equal Opportunity Employment report filed in 2014, sixty of eighty-three leadership positions at Apple were held by white men. At Facebook, 32 percent of workers are women, and women hold only 16 percent of their tech jobs and 23 percent of their leadership roles. Many have suggested that the gender disparity is caused in part by expectations that employees work long hours and weekends and that egg freezing both highlights and delays a larger problem: a workplace that does not make room for having and raising children. I see the value in these arguments, yet it's hard for me, as someone who had very limited insurance coverage while undergoing IVF, to look askance at any expansion of reproduction options.

If I had a younger sister who wondered if she should freeze her eggs while she waited for the right partner or the right moment in her life and career, I'd suggest she first see her gynecologist or a reproductive endocrinologist for a fertility workup. A simple blood test can give women and their doctors valuable information about ovarian reserve.

212 **It took five days of watching and waiting for the gorilla keepers to decide that enough was enough; they finally sedated Olympia and gave Bomassa back to Jamani:** Aaron Jesue emphasizes that it takes extensive training to build the gorillas' trust during medical and emergency procedures. He reports that Olympia actively participated in a hand injection during the sedation process.

SELECTED BIBLIOGRAPHY

Albee, Edward. *Who's Afraid of Virginia Woolf? A Play.* New York: Atheneum, 1962.

Association of Zoos and Aquariums. "Species Survival Plan (SSP) Programs." Accessed on September 13, 2015. https://www.aza.org /species-survival-plan-program/.

Atwood, Margaret. "Haunted by *The Handmaid's Tale.*" *Guardian,* January 20, 2012. http://www.theguardian.com/books/2012/jan /20/handmaids-tale-margaret-atwood.

"Baby M Grew Up, but Surrogacy Remains Controversial." *New York Times,* March 24, 2014. http://parenting.blogs.nytimes.com/2014 /03/24/baby-m-grew-up-but-surrogacy-remains-controversial/.

Begos, Kevin, and Danielle Deaver. *Against Their Will: North Carolina's Sterilization Program.* Apalachicola, FL: Gray Oak, 2012.

Bell, Ann V. "Beyond (Financial) Accessibility: Inequalities within the Medicalisation of Infertility." *Sociology of Health and Illness* 32, no. 4 (2010): 631–46.

Blankenhorn, David. "How My View on Gay Marriage Changed." *New York Times,* June 22, 2012.

Bleakney, Elaine. *For Another Writing Back.* Portland, OR: Sidebrow, 2014.

Brief of Gary J. Gates as Amicus Curiae on the Merits in Support of Respondent Windsor. United States v. Windsor, 570 U.S. ___ (2013), No. 12-307. http://www.glad.org/uploads/docs/cases/windsor-v -united-states/amicus-brief-of-gary-gates.pdf.

Brockwell, Holly. "Why Can't I Get Sterilised in My 20s?" *Guardian,* January 28, 2015. http://www.theguardian.com/commentisfree/ 2015/jan/28/why-wont-nhs-let-me-be-sterilised.

Brown, Lesley, and John Brown. *Our Miracle Called Louise: A Parents' Story.* New York: Paddington, 1979.

Case, Neko. "Hold On, Hold On." *Fox Confessor Brings the Flood.* ANTI- Records, 2006.

Ceballo, Rosario, Antonia Abbey, and Deborah Schooler. "Perceptions of Women's Infertility: What Do Physicians See?" *Fertility and Sterility* 93, no. 4 (2010): 1066–73.

Clarke, Edward H. *Sex in Education; or, A Fair Chance for the Girls.* Boston: J. R. Osgood, 1874.

Dickens, Charles. *Great Expectations.*

Didion, Joan. "The White Album." In *The White Album.* New York: Simon and Schuster, 1979.

Didion, Joan. *Blue Nights.* New York: Knopf, 2011.

Digby, Leslie J., and Stephen F. Ferrari. "Multiple Breeding Females in Free-Ranging Groups of *Callithrix jacchus.*" *International Journal of Primatology* 15, no. 3 (1994).

Digby, Leslie. "Infant Care, Infanticide, and Female Reproductive Strategies in Polygynous Groups of Common Marmosets *(Callithrix jacchus).*" *Behavioral Ecology and Sociobiology* 37, no. 1 (1995): 51–61.

Dinkin, Roxane Head, and Robert J. Dinkin. *Infertility and the Creative Spirit.* Bloomington, IN: iUniverse, 2011.

Donum Vitae: Instruction on Respect for Human Life in Its Origin and on the Dignity of Procreation. Vatican City: Congregation for the Doctrine of the Faith, 1987.

Edwards, Robert G. "The Bumpy Road to Human In Vitro Fertilization." *Nature Medicine* 7, no. 10 (2001): 1091–94. http://www.nature.com /nm/journal/v7/n10/full/nm1001-1091.html.

Ehrlich, Paul R. *The Population Bomb.* New York: Ballantine, 1968.

Ertman, Martha M. *Love's Promises: How Formal and Informal Contracts Shape All Kinds of Families.* Boston: Beacon, 2015.

Family Equality Council. "Non-Discrimination Laws." Accessed September 13, 2015. http://www.familyequality.org/get_informed /equality_maps/non-discrimination_laws/.

Flinn, Susan. "Lupron—What Does It Do to Women's Health?" *National Women's Health Network Newsletter,* September 1, 2008.

Google Baby. Directed by Zippi Brand Frank. Brandcom Productions and HBO Documentary Films, 2009.

Governor's Task Force to Determine the Method of Compensation for Victims of North Carolina's Eugenics Board. "Preliminary Report to

the Governor of the State of North Carolina." August 1, 2011. http://
www.sterilizationvictims.nc.gov/documents/preliminary_report.pdf.

Greenfield, Rebecca. "Sex-Crazed Cicadas Will Soon Outnumber
Humans 600-to-1." *The Wire,* May 6, 2013. http://www.thewire
.com/national/2013/05/cicada-to-human-ratio-2013/64933/.

Gussow, Mel. *Edward Albee: A Singular Journey; A Biography.* New
York: Simon and Schuster, 1999.

Haberman, Clyde. "Baby M and the Question of Surrogate Motherhood."
New York Times, March 23, 2014. http://www.nytimes.com/2014/03
/24/us/baby-m-and-the-question-of-surrogate-motherhood.html.

Harris, Emily. "Israeli Dads Welcome Surrogate-Born Baby in Nepal
on Earthquake Day." *All Things Considered.* NPR, April 29, 2015.

Hawkins, Jim. "Selling ART: An Empirical Assessment of Advertising
on Fertility Clinics' Websites." *Indiana Law Journal* 88 (2013):
1147–79.

Head, Jonathan. "Thailand Bans Commercial Surrogacy for Foreigners."
BBC News, February 20, 2015. http://www.bbc.com/news/world
-asia-31546717.

Hrdy, Sarah Blaffer. *Mother Nature: A History of Mothers, Infants, and
Natural Selection.* New York: Pantheon, 1999.

Hrdy, Sarah Blaffer. *Mothers and Others: The Evolutionary Origins of
Mutual Understanding.* Cambridge, MA: Belknap, 2009.

Kamin, Debra. "Israel Evacuates Surrogate Babies from Nepal but
Leaves the Mothers Behind." *Time,* April 28, 2015.

Kelly, Mike. "25 Years after Baby M, Surrogacy Questions Remain
Unanswered." *Bergen County Record,* March 30, 2012. http://www
.northjersey.com/news/kelly-25-years-after-baby-m-surrogacy
-questions-remain-unanswered-1.745725.

Kopsa, Andy. "State-Sanctioned Rape: Trans-Vaginal Ultrasound Laws
in Virginia, Texas, and Iowa." *RH Reality Check,* February 15, 2012.
http://rhrealitycheck.org/article/2012/02/15/government
-sanctioned-rape-in-state-virginia-and-texas/.

Lerner, Ben. *10:04: A Novel.* New York: Faber and Faber, 2014.

Lunenfeld, Bruno. "Historical Perspectives in Gonadotropin Therapy."
Human Reproduction Update 10, no. 6 (2004): 453–67.

Maxwell, William. *So Long, See You Tomorrow.* New York: Knopf, 1980.

May, Elaine Tyler. *Barren in the Promised Land: Childless Americans
and the Pursuit of Happiness.* New York: Basic Books, 1995.

Mead, Rebecca. "Cold Comfort: Tech Jobs and Egg Freezing." *New*

Yorker, October 17, 2014. http://www.newyorker.com/news/daily
-comment/facebook-apple-egg-freezing-benefits.

Molinaro, Thomas. "One or Two? The Debate on Single Embryo
Transfer." Reproductive Medicine Associates of New Jersey,
January 3, 2014. http://www.rmanj.com/2014/01/one-two
-debate-single-embryo-transfer/.

Morgan, Lynn. *Icons of Life: A Cultural History of Human Embryos.*
Oakland, CA: Univ. of California Press, 2009.

Morrison, Toni. *Sula.* New York: Knopf, 1974.

Morrison, Toni. *Beloved: A Novel.* New York: Knopf, 1987.

NeJaime, Douglas. "*Griswold*'s Progeny: Assisted Reproduction,
Procreative Liberty, and Sexual Orientation Equality." Forum. *Yale
Law Journal* 124 (2015): 340. http://papers.ssrn.com/sol3/papers.
cfm?abstract_id=2579409.

North Carolina Zoo. "Zoo Loses Male Gorilla 'Nkosi.'" September 3,
2013. http://www.nczoo.org/Newsroom.aspx?pageID=12643&CNM
=undefined&contentPage=true&desc=false&listingID=184#.

Obergefell v. Hodges, 576 U.S. ___ (2015), No. 14-556.

Olsen, Tillie. *Silences.* 1st Feminist Press ed. New York: Feminist Press
at the City Univ. of New York, 2003.

Ombelet, Willem, and Johan Van Robays. "History of Human Artificial
Insemination." In *Artificial Insemination: An Update,* monograph.
Edited by Willem Ombelet and Herman Tournaye. *Facts, Views
and Vision in Obstetrics and Gynaecology* (2010): 1–5. http://www
.researchgate.net/publication/228363363_History_of_human
_artificial_insemination.

Parsons, Sabrina. "Female Tech CEO: Egg-Freezing 'Benefit' Sends
the Wrong Message to Women." *Business Insider,* October 20, 2014.
http://www.businessinsider.com/apple-facebook-egg-freezing
-benefit-is-bad-for-women-2014-10#ixzz3k1iuI5mm.

Petersen, Melody. "2 Drug Makers to Pay $875 Million to Settle Fraud
Case." *New York Times,* October 4, 2001.

Peterson, Iver. "Fitness Test for Baby M's Mother Unfair, Feminists
Say." *New York Times,* March 20, 1987. http://www.nytimes.com
/1987/03/20/nyregion/fitness-test-for-baby-m-s-mother-unfair
-feminists-say.html.

Railey, John. *Rage to Redemption in the Sterilization Age: A
Confrontation with American Genocide.* Eugene, OR: Cascade
Books, 2015.

Raising Arizona. Directed by Joel and Ethan Coen. Circle Films, 1987.

Rich, Adrienne. *Of Woman Born: Motherhood as Experience and Institution.* New York: Norton, 1976.

Roe v. Wade, 410 U.S. 113 (1973).

Rosner, Marni. "Recovery from Traumatic Loss: A Study of Women Living without Children after Infertility." Doctorate in social work (DSW) diss., Univ. of Pennsylvania, 2012. Paper 20. http://repository.upenn.edu/edissertations_sp2/20.

Rotkirch, Anna. "'All That She Wants Is A(nother) Baby'? Longing for Children as a Fertility Incentive of Growing Importance." *Journal of Evolutionary Psychology* 5, no. 1 (2007): 89–104.

Rotkirch, Anna. "What Is 'Baby Fever'? Contrasting Evolutionary Explanations of Proceptive Behavior." *The New Evolutionary Social Science: Human Nature, Social Behavior, and Social Change.* Edited by Hans-Jürgen Niedenzu, Tamás Meleghy, and Peter Meyer. Boulder, CO: Paradigm, 2008.

Sartin, Jeffrey S. "J. Marion Sims, the Father of Gynecology: Hero or Villain?" *Southern Medical Journal* 97, no. 5 (2004): 500–505.

Schwartz, Barry. *The Paradox of Choice: Why More Is Less.* New York: Ecco, 2004.

Senior, Jennifer. *All Joy and No Fun: The Paradox of Modern Parenthood.* New York: Ecco/HarperCollins, 2014.

Shakespeare, William. *Macbeth.* Annotated and with an introduction by Burton Raffel. New Haven: Yale Univ. Press, 2005.

Solomon, Andrew. "Love, No Matter What." Filmed April 2013. TEDMED video, 23:27. http://www.ted.com/talks/andrew_solomon_love_no_matter_what.

Solomon, Andrew. *Far from the Tree: Parents, Children, and the Search for Identity.* New York: Scribner, 2012.

Steinbock, Bonnie. *Life before Birth: The Moral and Legal Status of Embryos and Fetuses.* New York: Oxford Univ. Press, 1992.

Sullivan, Mecca Jamilah. "A Magic of Bags." *Blue Talk and Love: Stories.* New York: Riverdale Avenue Books, 2015.

Thorton, Mary. "They Call Him . . . Saint." *Australian Women's Weekly,* March 9, 1966.

"Timeline: The History of In Vitro Fertilization." *American Experience* online. PBS. Accessed on September 12, 2015. http://www.pbs.org/wgbh/americanexperience/features/timeline/babies/.

Tran, Mark. "Apple and Facebook Offer to Freeze Eggs for Female

Employees." *Guardian,* October 15, 2014. http://www.theguardian
.com/technology/2014/oct/15/apple-facebook-offer-freeze-eggs
-female-employees.

Tulandi, Togas, Leonora King, and Phyllis Zelkowitz. "Public Funding
of and Access to In Vitro Fertilization." *New England Journal of
Medicine* 368, no. 20 (2013): 1948–49.

Woolf, Virginia. *Moments of Being: Unpublished Autobiographical
Writings.* Edited and with an introduction and notes by Jeanne
Schulkind. New York: Harcourt Brace Jovanovich, 1976.

Woolf, Virginia. "Lappin and Lapinova." In *The Virginia Woolf Reader.*
Edited by Mitchell Alexander Leaska. San Diego: Harcourt Brace
Jovanovich, 1984.

Zuk, Marlene. *Paleofantasy: What Evolution Really Tells Us about Sex,
Diet, and How We Live.* New York: W. W. Norton, 2014.

BELLE BOGGS is the author of *Mattaponi Queen,* a collection of linked stories set along Virginia's Mattaponi River. *Mattaponi Queen* won the Bakeless Prize and the Library of Virginia Literary Award, and was a finalist for the Frank O'Connor International Short Story Award. Boggs has received fellowships from the National Endowment for the Arts, the North Carolina Arts Council, and the Bread Loaf and Sewanee writers' conferences. Her stories and essays have appeared in the *Paris Review, Orion, Harper's, Glimmer Train, Slate, Ecotone,* the *Sun,* and other publications. She teaches in the MFA program at North Carolina State University.

The text of *The Art of Waiting* is set in Century Old Style. Book design and composition by Bookmobile Design & Digital Publisher Services, Minneapolis, Minnesota. Manufactured by Versa Press on acid-free, 30 percent postconsumer wastepaper.